chemo cookery club

Published by Metro Publishing
an imprint of John Blake Publishing Ltd,
3 Bramber Court, 2 Bramber Road,
London W14 9PB, England

www.johnblakepublishing.co.uk
www.facebook.com/Johnblakepub
twitter.com/johnblakepub

First published in paperback in 2013

ISBN: 978-1-78219-362-3

British Library Cataloguing-in-Publication Data:
A catalogue record for this book is available from
the British Library.

Printed and bound in China by
Toppan Leefung Printing Ltd

1 3 5 7 9 10 8 6 4 2

© Repertoire Food & Design Ltd.
Text Penny Ericson.
Design and photographs Simon Firullo

Papers used by John Blake Publishing are natural, recyclable
products made from wood grown in sustainable forests. The
manufacturing processes conform to the environmental
regulations of the country of origin.

acknowledgements

I've had wonderful help and guidance producing
Chemo Cookery Club. I'm a jackdaw when it comes
to recipes and have acquired this collection from
countless sources. There are a few I can take unique
credit for but I reckon even those have another source
of inspiration. Thanks to all the friends, family and
professionals whose recipes I have drawn upon and
been inspired by.

I owe thanks to so many for testing recipes, offering
themselves as guinea pigs and providing guidance,
support and input. I am especially grateful to the
patients and carers we've met along the way for ideas,
recipes and testimonials.

I owe a world of thanks to Mark Pollack & Ben
Delamere, Barbara Thomson, Karen Wells & all at
The Chestnut Horse, Jane Johnston & David Mairs,
Erica & Shawn O'Rourke, Chef Kate Hughes & all at
Cook Academy, Lesley & Stewart Carr, Juliet Alexander,
Stephen Cook & all at Walter Rose Butchers, Chef
Richard Skinner, everyone on C2 North Hampshire
County Hospital Basingstoke, everyone at Nick Jonas
Royal Hampshire County Hospital Winchester,
David Gard, Bill Reinking, Sandra MacDonald,
Karen Marinnan, Jane Aspell & Jim Mills, Stuart Daniel,
Josh & Fenella Fitch & all the little Fitchs. Finally, Phil
for stirring the pot and Peter for telling me just to
get on with it.

Special thanks to Jane Graham Maw of Graham Maw
Christie Literary Agency and everyone at John Blake
Publishing for believing in us.

Any errors are entirely mine.

chemo cookery club

over 150 delicious and healthy recipes
for your journey to recovery

Penny Ericson
Photographs Simon Firullo

metro

a note to our readers

Whilst I have worked very hard to ensure the recipes and contents of this book are nutritionally sound, everyone has individual needs. This book does not offer specific dietary advice, rather it is a collection of ideas for the people and their carers, whose health and treatment has affected the daily pleasures of food. If you have any questions about what is best or appropriate for you, consult your dietician or doctor.

Chemo Cookery Club has been produced, in its entirety, in domestic kitchens using domestic tools, appliances and utilities and the photography is a true representation of the dishes.

I haven't had the sophisticated and scientific conditions of a commercial kitchen. As such, things like cooking times and temperature controls may vary. The oven temperatures used are, °Cf, centigrade, fan-assisted, (see conversion chart, oven temperatures, page 278).

the principles about ingredients and preparation are simple:

My process has been 'market to table in a day'. This meant: shop, prep, cook, serve and eat in a single session. Each recipe is part of 'a day in the life' of someone either living on their own and undergoing treatment or a carer responsible for the well-being of someone in treatment of one form or another and treated in the manner that they would go about things. In other words not as professional chefs and medical professionals but as mere mortals with the resources we have to hand.

I believe in 'field-to-fork' by the quickest and closest route. I have used readily available ingredients from markets, butchers, farms, green grocers and supermarkets. The fresher the ingredients the higher their nutritional value, for example, potatoes straight from the field retain their full nutritional value whereas washed and bagged supermarket potatoes inevitably lose some of their value due to refrigeration, shipping and storage.

There are a few ingredients that I use that may not be familiar and a few others where I use a generic description but use a specific type or brand. They are:

pastry

I have chosen to use store bought short pastry, puff pastry and filo. Wherever possible the recipes are designed to ease complexity and deliver a great dish. This seemed like a natural shortcut.

sauces and marinades

Here I have offered a mixture, some from scratch, others store bought. For example, I have given a recipe for teriyaki marinade but you may find it easier to use store bought. Where I have included a recipe it's because the flavours are inherent to the dish. Store bought will alter the nutritional analysis as they tend to be higher in salt, sugar and kcals

'season to taste'

This generally means add salt and pepper to taste. When preparing dishes I season throughout the process as this produces a different flavour to seasoning only at the end of preparation.

pepper
This is black pepper unless specified otherwise, for example, white, freshly cracked or chilli.

salt
I have used Maldon sea salt unless otherwise specified. If this is unavailable, a delicate fleur de sel (also a fine sea salt) is a good substitute. Table salt can be sharper so be careful.

sriracha
Is a chilli sauce originally from Malaysia. Used judiciously it adds lift to sauces and marinades without the intense heat of other chilli sauces. It is great for bumping up flavour in response to loss of taste as the result of treatment. It is available in many supermarkets and Asian grocery stores. For a bit more information about chilli paste and seasoning with chillies go to 'the basics', page 284.

a word on wine, spirits and the use of alcohol
Some of the *Chemo Cookery Club* recipes include alcohol as an ingredient. It's used to add and enhance flavour, for example, in a marinade or flambé or as an aperitif to 'tingle the taste buds'. The intention is to encourage the enjoyment of food and find ways to enhance nutritional intake. Remember that, when heated, alcohol evaporates but the flavour remains, so it's not like you'll be glugging down half bottles of wine or anything like that!

In every instance the recipes can be followed without the use of alcohol. Substitutes can be used, for example using a juniper berry infusion to replace gin. I leave it to you, the cook, to choose.

In general, the advice about drinking alcohol after a cancer diagnosis is expressed in terms of whether you've been a drinker in the past or not. If you have not previously been a drinker at all then, best not to start! If you have enjoyed a glass or three though, it's recommended that you have alcohol-free days and try to keep to as little as possible when you do. Ideally no more than 1-2 units a day, as alcohol is known to increase the risk of a number of cancers.

Sound guidance and helpful information is available on the *World Cancer Research Fund* and *American Institute of Cancer Research* websites.

a word on shortcuts
The spirit of this book is to make good food accessible when times aren't their best. There are so many well-prepared foods available today. If you fancy a recipe but the preparation seems daunting go and buy it ready-made then do the easy stuff like preparing fresh sauces and condiments.

'I lost my mother to cancer several years ago and as a chef I increasingly find myself researching the preventative aspects of good nutrition through good food. Indeed, I created an entire restaurant cuisine around it. With internationally recognised bodies such as The *World Cancer Research Fund* providing irrefutable proof that food has a direct impact on cancer and its prevention, it can no longer be argued otherwise. Penny's original concept and recipes in this book go a long way to helping both sufferers and those who simply want great tasting food.'

Michelin starred Chef Chris Horridge

'Eating healthily can make such a valuable difference to your life. A healthy diet is one that gives you everything you need to keep your body working well. Eating well and keeping to a healthy weight will help you maintain or regain your strength, have more energy, and have an increased sense of well-being. During and after treatment for cancer, many people can experience eating problems. These can be related to the cancer itself, or the side effects of different treatments. If you're the main carer for someone with cancer, it can be upsetting and difficult to know how to deal with the eating problems their cancer or treatments have caused. But there are things people can do to help make eating easier and ensure they have adequate nutrition while having treatment. These can help both the person with cancer and their family and friends.'

Ciaran Devane, CEO, *MacMillan Cancer Support*

'We are delighted to be associated with The *Chemo Cookery Club Cookery book*. Enjoying food and eating nutritionally is often a struggle during illness and chemotherapy treatments. Penny's book provides an invaluable insight into our relationship with food during this time as well as practical advice on which foods are worth encouraging and permission to succumb to cravings from time to time.

Not only are the recipes easy to make using everyday ingredients but they are incredibly delicious. We hope that this book will be a source of inspiration and practical help for cancer patients and their carers.'

Sue Airey, Head of Clinical and Care Services at *Bowel Cancer UK*

contents

introduction   13

    about our thumbs-up & nutritional analysis   15

    some sound principles & helpful hints   16

    your new best friends   17

off to a great start   24

grazing   48

soups   72

salads   98

pizza, pasta & risotto   120

vegetables & side dishes   144

fish & shellfish   174

poultry & game   200

beef, lamb, pork & venison   224

sweeties   246

for our international friends

    conversion chart   278

    the basics   280

    glossary of terms   283

index   284

'Going through chemotherapy can be a traumatic time and treatment can have side effects like loss of appetite and mouth ulcers, making it difficult to eat and enjoy food. This book could make the difference between patients eating and not eating; giving them and their families the tools to make delicious meals.'

Mark Flannagan, CEO, *Beating Bowel Cancer*

'The *Pelican Cancer Foundation* works to cure and improve the quality of life for patients with pelvic area and liver cancer through advancing the techniques of precision surgery and treatment, supporting research and sharing life-saving and life-enhancing knowledge and skills with cancer surgeons and specialists across the UK. Nutrition is an essential part of the recovery process and we are delighted to be associated with *Chemo Cookery Club*. This book gives cancer patients and their carers some great ideas on how to make food exciting and irresistible.'

Sarah Crane, CEO, *Pelican Cancer Foundation*

introduction

Chemo Cookery Club is not about making special food. It's about making food special. Turning lemons into lemonade.

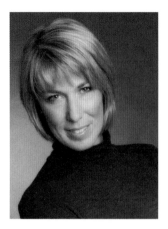

Following a fund-raising charity book Simon and I published, *Polo Picnic*, in aid of the Helen Reinking Trust for Alzheimer's Society, a friend suggested I do something similar for cancer patients and carers. I assumed there would be plenty of cookbooks out there already. I then considered the particular expertise required to do the job and decided I wasn't qualified. I'm not a doctor or a dietician. I'm not even a chef! I crumpled up the notion and filed it in the 'too difficult' bin.

Then I met a guy in my local pub who made me think again. About a lot of things actually. He was midway through a course of chemotherapy following the removal of a malignant tumour the size of a grapefruit from his colon six months earlier. We got talking. His positive attitude was contagious. But it was clear he had been given little in the way of dietary information to help him through his treatment and recovery.

This got me thinking. I don't know anyone who hasn't been touched by chronic and debilitating illnesses such as cancer, Crohn's or diabetes in some way. I've experienced all three in my life, as patient, daughter, friend and now wife to that guy in the pub. So I decided that being a published and skilled cook and carer was enough qualification. I could get professional advice from the experts.

I started by searching for books with a joyful view of food and an appreciation of the special circumstances of patients who experience things like 'rubber mouth' and 'metal mouth'. Books that didn't look and feel like the inside of a clinic. I couldn't find any. They just weren't there.

It was a steep learning curve. You don't think of chemo suites as being especially foodie but I was soon to realise that food was foremost in people's minds, especially those plonked into the role of carer for the first time. All too often I heard stories from people who had little experience of preparing family meals or managing the weekly shopping. Chopping an onion could be far more intimidating than executing mega-deals in the boardroom. Listening to so many stories of how the enjoyment of food could be turned upside down or, discovered anew, from so many gave me great inspiration.

Wellness isn't just about diet. It's also about how we feel and satisfy our desires. We eat with our eyes. My creative partner and friend of many years, Simon Firullo's photography and design have made this book a thing of mouth-watering beauty.

I hope *Chemo Cookery Club* inspires those surviving illness and their loved ones to treat the experience of preparing and enjoying food as a part of wellness. We all need to eat, even when we don't feel our best. I hope these recipes bring comfort and happiness. Enjoy!

Penny

'*Oracle Cancer Trust* strives to ensure that we preserve the delicate senses so often affected by the treatment for head and neck cancers and we are delighted to be associated with *Chemo Cookery Club* which offers such a wonderful support to cancer patients and their carers, enhancing their quality of life through the enjoyment of food.'

Amanda Croft-Pearman, COO, *Oracle Cancer Trust*

'Eating a balanced and varied diet can help some people cope with breast cancer and its treatments. Chemotherapy can affect a person's appetite as a result of side effects such as nausea, a sore mouth or taste changes. At *Breast Cancer Care*, we know how much people can value quick, simple recipes, with flavourful foods that are easy and enjoyable to eat.'

Emma Pennery, Director of Clinical Services at *Breast Cancer Care*

about our thumbs-up nutritional analysis

In providing the nutritional values of our recipes we use purpose built software called, Dietplan (version 6). The recipe analyses have been carried out by Barbara Parry, MSc RD, senior research dietician in the Winchester and Andover Breast Unit at the Royal Hampshire County Hospital, Winchester, UK. She has been a registered dietician since 1982 and a specialist diet and breast cancer researcher since 1996.

The information is intended as general guidance, not as clinical research or medical advice. There are too many variables regarding the source of ingredients, age and quality to be perfectly accurate.

For detailed information regarding specific foods and ingredients two good sources of information are: the *World Cancer Research Fund*, www.wcrf-uk.org and the *American Institute for Cancer Research*. www.aicr.org. If you require specific advice contact your doctor or registered dietician.

about the thumbs-up scores

The nutritional analysis uses a generous point of reference. The 'thumbs-up' scoring for recipes is based on a percentage of, 'Reference Nutrition Intake, RNI', based on a number of general assumptions. Everyone's nutritional requirements are different, so I wanted to give you confidence that the recipes are good sources of these nutrients and also give consistency.

My husband and chief guinea pig, Simon was chosen as the 'standard person' to base the RNI comparisons on. He's a 50-ish male of moderate occupational and recreational activity. Male RNI's are generally higher for nutrients than the female equivalent and this offers an approximation for any increased energy needs that people undergoing treatment might have. As the RNI for iron is generally higher for women than men, an average of the male and female RNI's have been used for comparing iron contributions of the recipes.

Special provision has not been made for children in the nutritional analysis but that is not to say these recipes might not tempt the tastebuds of any age.

If a particular nutrient isn't listed beside a recipe, this doesn't mean the recipe is necessarily devoid of that nutrient, just that a portion provides less than 20% of the RNI (and so doesn't have a thumbs-up equivalent). The thumbs-up scoring is based on:

>100%	>👍👍👍👍
80-100%	👍👍👍👍
60-79%	👍👍👍
40-59%	👍👍
20-39%	👍

1-19% nil but may at times be credited for other value

The RNI is the amount of a nutrient that is enough to ensure that the needs of nearly all the population (97.5%) are being met. Individual nutritional needs vary widely. Our figures are based on the UK population, not individuals. For further information about RNI visit www.foodafactoflife.org.uk.

Our recipes may contain some ingredients that, during your treatment, you've been advised to avoid by your specialists. We recommend that you follow this advice. The recipes do lend themselves to substituting ingredients (even though this will change the nutrient analysis somewhat) and we encourage you to do this to make a recipe just right for you.

some sound principles and helpful hints

positive associations

We enjoy food with all our senses so if one or two of them aren't working at optimum strength it helps to enhance the experience of the others. It's been said that we eat with our eyes. If you can, take time and make dishes beautiful. Allow aromas to fill the room. How often have we heard comfort associated with the smell of baked bread or bacon frying in a pan?

Get to know your high days and low days. Our memories can play powerful tricks. When you can, plan your menus so that you have your favourite meals when you are feeling well. Have simple foods on and just after treatment days. Enjoy them with loved ones and friends.

Succumb to your cravings. Your body might be telling you that you need something. Don't break the rules; if you crave chocolate and aren't meant to have it, think what it's rich in, such as potassium and try a banana instead. Variety and small portions taken regularly can help ward off nausea and fatigue.

get ready

There are a few things you can do to smooth the way if you have time. Such as:

- go to the dentist before treatment begins

- adjust your wardrobe so you have clothes that are comfortable and easy to get in and out of

- plan how your laundry will be done if you won't feel up to doing it

- arrange the rooms where you will spend most of your time so that they are easy to move around and have what you want, for example, a supply of bottled water next to the bed. Make them rooms you want to spend time in

- stock the loo with plenty of supplies like toothpaste, loo roll, towels, facecloths and air freshener

- remove temptation – clear out and restock the kitchen cupboards and fridge

- stock up on food and supplies you know you will need and enjoy. For example, pre-freeze fresh fruit for smoothies

- find out who your best support groups are for things like hair-loss and carers support

Some kitchen tools that are endlessly useful are a high-powered blender, food processor, hand blender and a slow cooker. A good supply of cling film and freezer bags and small storage containers are also good to have to hand.

When I began writing this book I wasn't surprised by the amount of nutritional information and advice available. It is literally everywhere. I was overwhelmed by the amount of conflicting opinions and contradictory published research. What I wanted to know first and foremost was which foods could I rely on to be known as helpful, healthy and in some cases cancer arresting and preventative. With that I could use those foods as the foundation for the recipes. I needed an expert.

Fortune favoured me. Simon was undergoing his second tour of chemo in the 'Nick Jonas Cancer Day Ward' at the Royal Hampshire Hospital in Winchester. He willingly agreed to donate his biopsies and related tests and treatment results to research at the hospital and the Pelican Foundation. Through this we learned that an experienced cancer research dietician was right on our doorstep.

Chemo Cookery Club really came alive the day I met Barbara Parry, MSc RD, in her crowded wee office tucked in a remote corner of the hospital. It soon became clear that she shared my view that everyday foods could be important sources of nutrition for people undergoing treatment and that such foods can mean more to people after a cancer diagnosis than just the nutrients they might provide. Everyday foods and recipes could make a difference to people during a time of so much upheaval and change. I made a wonderful friend that day.

Barbara has brought so much to this project. We affectionately call her contribution, 'the science bits' and without them this would be just another recipe book. These are the 'bits' that give the book nutritional reliability and gravitas.

So here are some of Barbara's thoughts on the ingredients we highlight in this book, based on her years of experience as a registered dietitian working in research, health promotion, clinical dietetics and her collaborations with colleagues within the global network of cancer research organisations.

your new best friends — 'make these a few of your favourite things' by Barbara Parry, MSc RD

Wouldn't it be grand if food could prevent or cure cancer! Alas, this is not so – YET.

The right food can, however, lower the risk of developing the disease, aid in treatment and recovery – physically, mentally and emotionally. Many foods have cancer-fighting properties such as antioxidants and we are beginning to understand how phytochemical compounds protect cells from disease.

Cancer does not manifest overnight. It takes time to develop and goes through stages. We know good eating and a healthy diet can be of great assistance to the quality of life during all stages of cancer and it's many forms of treatment and after. There is also extensive and compelling evidence that certain foods and preparation methods can contribute to cancer developing and most importantly in the prevention of it.

Initiation, promotion, progression, actual and metastasis (spread) are the stages. Get to know them and learn as much as you can about where you are and how nutrition can help.

Don't forget, we eat with our eyes. In many instances the best nutrition comes from the very components that give food its colour. It seems nature intended wellness to be bold and bright!

Whenever possible, choose foods that are in season and as fresh as they possibly can be. Locally sourced foods have often travelled shorter distances from field-to-shopping basket and so may be better sources of nutrients, particularly if prepared in a way that will preserve those water-soluble and heat sensitive ones.

It might be helpful to include a probiotic supplement if your treatment results in digestive problems such as diarrhoea and abdominal discomfort as a result of flatulence. Probiotics are a source of 'friendly bacteria' that can help replace the natural bacteria in your gut and aid digestion. Be mindful that treatment can reduce your white blood cell count, known as neutropenia and if so, you may be advised to avoid foods and drinks (including probiotics, live and bio products, uncooked foods, even ordinary tap water) to reduce your risk of developing a food- or water-borne infection. Remember, the definitive guide is always best to come from a registered dietician or your doctor.

Here are a few of the foods that are highlighted in this book that have been shown to be beneficial.

Make them your new best friends!

alliums — garlic & onions, leek & chives
Alliums are truly amazing vegetables. Laboratory studies show that they contain compounds that can help slow or stop tumour cell growth and these vegetables continue to be studied for their protective effects against cancers.

We're gradually learning how even the humble onion can be a dietary super hero. It's already a great ingredient that features in many of *Chemo Cookery Club*'s recipes alongside its cousins, garlic and leeks.

avocados
Just one avocado contains one quarter of the adult recommended daily amount of potassium and provides a rich source of a number of nutrients that can act as antioxidants and attack free radicals in the body. Guacamole is an easy and light snack anytime.

beans — legumes & pulses
Lentils, peas, chickpeas, soya, fava and unlimited varieties are full of phytochemicals found naturally in plants. They are also a great source of fibre that helps our digestive system get rid of waste efficiently, including things that may be harmful to our health. This is one of the reasons why beans and other fibre rich foods are associated with a reduced risk of bowel cancer. Beans are also a great source of protein and a really good source of iron (especially when eaten with foods or drinks that are a good source of vitamin C; vitamin C enhances the absorption of iron from plant foods). Soya beans in particular contain 'isoflavones' which are naturally occurring oestrogen-like chemicals that may block breast tumour growth. Lentils and peas are wonderfully versatile and full of flavour. Chickpeas make a great snack as they come or made into hummus.

beetroot
Beetroot and other purple foods such as red cabbage, aubergine and red grapes contain

anthocyanins that have been shown in laboratory studies to kill cancer cells and fight blood related cancers. They are also rich in cancer-fighting flavonoids. After you've eaten a lot of beetroot, don't be alarmed if your wee turns pink! Add beetroot to salads or make a visually stunning beetroot risotto. Yummy.

berries

Like beetroot, berries are colourful fruits, that are high in fibre and vitamin C, and there are so many varieties to enjoy – cherries, cranberries, raspberries, blackberries, blueberries, strawberries, damsons, loganberries, tayberries...the list goes on! Great eaten on their own or added to brighten a meal. How much more delicious is the simplest of fruit salads thanks to the addition of a handful of colourful berries. Start the day with a berry smoothie and round off the weekend with a mixed-berry topped pavlova or freeze grapes and use them as ice cubes.

carrots

Carrots are orange in colour because of the β-carotene they contain; β-carotene is one of a group of naturally occurring chemicals called 'carotenoids' which are antioxidants. Raw carrots are also a source of 'falcarinol' that researchers suggest may slow the growth of cancer cells. Carrots are super as a snack on their own. They are also marvellous julienned and added to any stir-fry as they hold their shape and texture and add the perfect contrast to a green medley. Apricots, squash and sweet potatoes are also a good source of carotenoids. Orange just became one of my favourite colours!

cruciferous vegetables – broccoli, brussels sprouts, bok choi, cabbage, cauliflower & kale

These beautiful vegetables contain chemicals called 'glucosinolates' that, when digested are broken down into isothiocyanates and indoles. In laboratory and human studies, all of these are demonstrating beneficial effects for cancer prevention.

Raw broccoli is higher in calcium and vitamins A and C than milk and oranges. As we usually eat broccoli cooked, the heat sensitive and water-soluble nutrients such as vitamin C and calcium can be diminished. We are still learning how powerful these wonderful veggies truly are. Make a batch of cauliflower and cumin soup and stick small portions in the freezer for light meals. Try a broccoli purée with baked salmon or just munch fresh and raw with tzatziki and hummus. Delicious.

organic eggs & egg yolk

Eggs provide us with the highest quality dietary protein, most readily providing us with essential amino acids that our bodies aren't able to manufacture. The fat profile of eggs varies according to the diet of the hens that lay them. The fat is found exclusively in the yolk. Eggs are also a good source of folic acid and riboflavin (B-group vitamins) as well as the antioxidant trace mineral, selenium.

Soufflés and fluffy omelettes are a lovely way to enjoy eggs. They can be either savoury or sweet and are easy to eat and digest.

mushrooms

Mushrooms are a particularly good source of the B-vitamins, riboflavin, niacin and pantothenic acid as well as the minerals copper and selenium. Some people just can't get their heads around the texture of mushrooms. If you are one of them, try not to pass the little belters by. Added as a purée to sauces they don't have to overpower other ingredients and all the goodness is still there.

oily fish & flaxseed

As a source of omega-3 fats these are unequalled. Oily fish such as herring, mackerel and salmon are important sources of vitamin A, selenium and vitamin D as well as omega-3 fats. Oily fish (in fact, fish in general) is also a good source of protein and naturally low in saturated fats.

Worldwide there are concerns about the toxins that can accumulate in fish that result from the pollution of our oceans and rivers. Heavy metal toxicity, eg mercury, is a particular concern. Further, certain fishing methods are environmentally destructive which may discourage us from choosing fish as part of our regular eating pattern. Take care in sourcing your fish and shellfish; buy from stockists that have a clear sustainability policy.

We have been advised for many years to include oily fish 2-3 times per week for a healthy heart and to reduce risk of stroke but it is emerging as important for cancer prevention as well. The omega-3 fats have been shown through laboratory studies to reduce inflammation and encourage the synthesis of prostaglandins; both processes which disrupt the survival of cancer cells.

Salmon from well-managed fisheries, sardines, farmed rainbow trout, barramundi, farmed mussels and other shellfish are less likely to have high levels of environmental toxins but it is always a good idea to ask your fish supplier for more information.

Flaxseed is the best plant source of omega 3 fats but the jury is still out as to whether it has an important role to play in cancer prevention. While it can boost your intake of magnesium, manganese, selenium, thiamine (vitamin B1) and dietary fibre, it may also interfere with the absorption of some medicines. Using 1-4 tablespoons per day appears to be safe but really it is probably 'one to watch' until more is known about its biological effects.

peppers & jalapenos

Peppers (capsicums) are a top source of vitamin C, especially when eaten raw. Chilli peppers such as jalapenos contain a chemical called capsaicin that is being studied further as it has been shown to kill prostate and lung cancer cells in laboratory studies. Capsaicin is the very ingredient that makes chillies hot and might be just the thing to give a zing to your tastebuds during treatment.

seeds & nuts

seeds and nuts such as pumpkin, sunflower and sesame seeds, almonds and walnuts are the most concentrated sources of plant protein and also contain other nutritional 'goodies' such as potassium, magnesium, zinc, vitamin E, iron, B vitamins and dietary fibre.

Zinc helps vitamin C do its job so healthy levels can improve healing time. Zinc also plays an important role in how well our tastebuds work (we lose our taste sensitivity if we become deficient in zinc) so enjoying foods that provide us with zinc could help tantalise a flagging appetite too. Some seeds and nuts can be a non-dairy source of calcium as well.

Being such a powerhouse of nutrition (after all, seeds can be the source of many a thriving new plant in the vegetable garden), they can boost your intake of nutrients even when only small amounts are eaten. While some people argue that peanuts are not truly nuts, peanut butter has to be one of the best comfort foods that delivers so much in such a friendly way. Have it on toast or try it with sliced banana in a sandwich...really!

spices — turmeric & pepper — the good ones

Whilst there is no definitive opinion on the curative properties of herbs and spices, the practice of using them as treatment goes back millennia and exists today in every culture. If for no other reason, herbs and spices give us flavour, texture and aroma. Good news for curry fans.

Chemo Cookery Club and its recipes use spices to delight the tastebuds. They are used in small quantities so we have chosen not to focus on their medicinal potential.

spinach & watercress

Dark green, leafy vegetables are great sources of dietary fibre, folate and carotenoids, all with potential cancer fighting properties. Perhaps it's the folate they contain that makes them most interesting. Folate is important for producing and maintaining healthy DNA that carries each cell's reproduction code. An error in the code means a mistake in the healthy division and reproduction of cells that may start the cancer process in the body.

Watercress is a rich source of the glucosinolate, gluconasturtiin (phenethylglucosinolate) and is allied to the cruciferous best friends we referred to earlier. Research is gradually helping us to understand why diets rich in such vegetables actually lowers cancer risk. As recently as last year, for example, an extract of watercress has been shown to disrupt the process by which breast cancer cells maintain their nutrition and blood supply. Without nutrients and blood to carry oxygen to them, cancer cells can't survive or reproduce, which is great news.

tomatoes

Tomatoes are rich in lycopene, an antioxidant that tackles those free radicals that are thought to trigger cancerous cell growth. Also found in some other vegetables and fruits, lycopene is actually best absorbed after cooking and is the most potent carotenoid antioxidant. Studies have shown lycopene to improve immune function, reduce inflammation and proliferation of cancer cells and even lower LDL ('bad') cholesterol.

Tomatoes are also rich in vitamin C, which is most abundant when raw. As variety is the spice of life, enjoy tomatoes raw, cooked and often.

water

Well, it isn't exactly food but it cannot be ignored. Dehydration is an often overlooked symptom and relief is easy. Drink as much as you can. Little and often. Flavour it, chill it, freeze it. Keep it with you.

whole grain

Perhaps a good place to start is by describing just what is meant by whole grain. There are three distinct parts to plant grains; the germ, containing vitamin E and other antioxidant nutrients plus some fat; the endosperm, containing predominantly starchy carbohydrate with some B vitamins and some protein; the bran, a potent source of dietary fibre and other vitamins, minerals and nutrients, many with antioxidants.

Whole grain and wholemeal are terms that we sometimes used interchangeably but when it comes to the type of bread we buy or bake, we tend to think of whole grain as a granary-type while wholemeal is the smooth one! Granary bread is not to everyone's taste but you'll still find the wholemeal varieties make a superior contribution to your nutrition than a white loaf. Having said that, a plain old white loaf has its place, especially if things are delicate in the colo-rectal department.

Whole grains are known to play an important role in prevention of cancers of the lower digestive tract and research continues to demonstrate cancer specific and other health benefits. Enjoy any grain-derived food whether it be a variety of bread, breakfast cereal, starchy grain, like rice, polenta or pasta and favour those labeled wholemeal or whole grain whenever you can for an extra boost to your nutrient intake. Whole grains are a great source of iron and B vitamins as well.

yoghurt & probiotics

Yoghurt is a light, nutrient-packed food that's so versatile it can be used in the main course then again for dessert! You can 'turn down the heat' in a curry by adding natural yoghurt but 'turn up the nutrition' because it's a great source of calcium, protein, B-group vitamins and can also be a source of 'friendly' bacteria.

A side effect of treatment can be disruption to the normal balance of 'friendly bacteria' in the digestive tract causing such problems as bloating, flatulence, abdominal cramps or diarrhoea. While everyone's mix of digestive bacteria is different, it's important to maintain the balance for healthy digestion and absorption of nutrients and to form part of the 'first line of defence' to protect the body from disease.

The Food and Agriculture Organisation/World Health Organisation definition states that probiotics are 'live micro-organisms which when administered in adequate amounts confer a health benefit on the host'. From a dietary point of view, to be labelled 'probiotic' a food must contain a live, 'viable', strain of cells with known health benefits. Research into probiotics has focused on groups of diseased subjects and positive benefits in healthy populations have been difficult to demonstrate. Studies continue to define the action of probiotics, however, suggest some potential benefits in the regulation of the inflammatory response in cells, protection against absorption of 'unfriendly' micro-organisms and a possible role in increasing the activity of 'natural killer cells', thereby potentially protecting against abnormal tumour cell growth.

Cautionary advice may be given recommending the avoidance of 'live' yoghurts if your white blood cell count is low (known as 'neutropenia'), Remember, the definitive guide is best to come from a registered dietician or your doctor.

In the absence of advice to the contrary, do try a delicious fruit smoothie to start your day. It's a great way to start the day when your appetite for solid food might be lacking.

for further information

A reliable website for further information is www.aicr.org, compiled by the American Institute for Cancer Research, as sister organisation to the UK-based charity, the World Cancer Research Fund. This website provides practical, evidence-based information about foods and all their wonderful constituents that research is constantly showing are beneficial for cancer prevention and more recently their emerging role in enhancing the outcomes of cancer treatment.

I am always coming up with new ideas and recipes and am already working on *Chemo Cookery Club* II! I have not just written this book and left you to your own devices, I've set up an online support section for you at www.chemocookeryclub.com where you can:

🍃 seek expert advice about food and nutrition

🍃 ask for a special recipe. Just submit the ingredients, I'll provide you with a delicious recipe

🍃 be kept informed about events we'll be holding throughout the year

🍃 comment on the the book and its contents and make suggestions

🍃 seek suppliers and organisations that get our thumbs-up

🍃 try out new recipes. I'm adding to the list daily and take requests. All recipes are given thumbs-up analysis

🍃 have your favourite recipe checked and analysed. Just submit it and we will send you back the thumbs-up score

🍃 visit our forum to ask advice or just communicate with other like-minded people.

I am always pleased to here from you and please feel free to email me at penny.ericson@chemocanteen.co.uk.

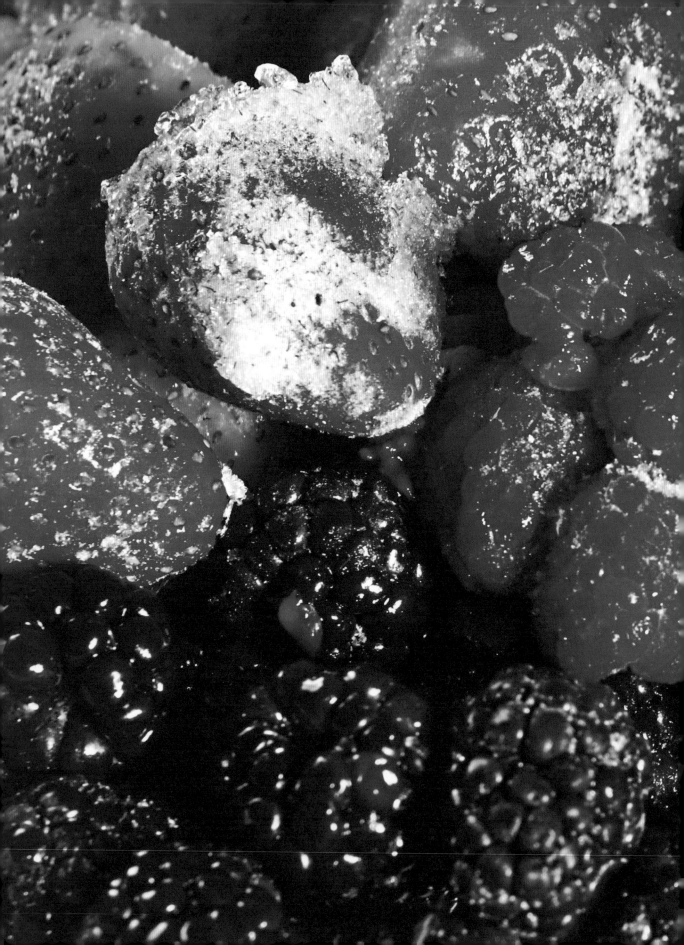

off to a great start

off to a great start

drinks, smoothies & shakes   28

    very berry breakfast smoothie   28

    frozen grapes in juice   30

    fruit juice ice cubes in yoghurt   31

    pineapple & ginger sherbet   32

    mango smoothie   32

    crème de menthe & chocolate frippery   35

    chocolate banana smoothie   35

    blueberry & yoghurt whippie   36

bacon & egger   39

old-fashioned french toast   40

perfect poached eggs with beans on toast   41

cheese soufflé   42

savoury egg cupcakes   45

waffles   46

crêpes   47

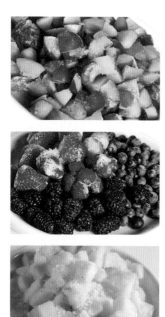

smoothies & shakes

The method is basic and the flavour combinations infinite. Chuck everything into a blender and whip until smooth. Voila!

If you want a creamier smoothie use more yoghurt and if you want to adjust the thickness use ice. If you want a creamy shake, use frozen yoghurt or ice cream (the nutritional values will vary somewhat). Pre-freezing the fruit also helps keep a thick and creamy consistency.

If you are sensitive to roughage such as seeds, piths and skins, once liquidised, pass through a sieve.

All of these mixtures can be frozen in ice cube trays or lolly moulds to make small snacks. They can be soothing on dry and tender mouths and also act as an appetite stimulant.

very berry breakfast smoothie
serves 2 full or 4 light portions

This is my favourite smoothie and a great way to start the day. For the berries I think the best combination is raspberries, blackberries, blueberries and currants.

nutrient	thumbs-up score
vitamin C	>👍👍👍👍
vitamin B6	>👍👍👍👍
calcium	👍👍
fibre	👍👍
(non-starch polysaccaride)	
phosphorus	👍👍
iodine	👍👍
folate	👍👍
potassium	👍👍
magnesium	👍
iron	👍
copper	👍
thiamin	👍
riboflavin	👍
protein	👍

100g yoghurt
250ml mixed apple & cranberry juice
1 slice pineapple, skin & eyes removed*
1 cup frozen mixed berries
½ cup strawberries

Each portion provides 9g protein and 320kcals

*see *the basics*, page 281

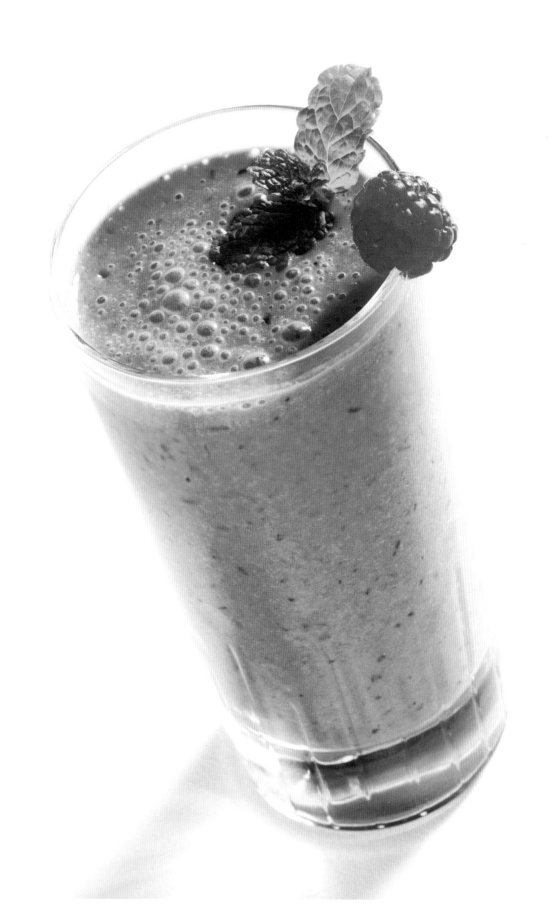

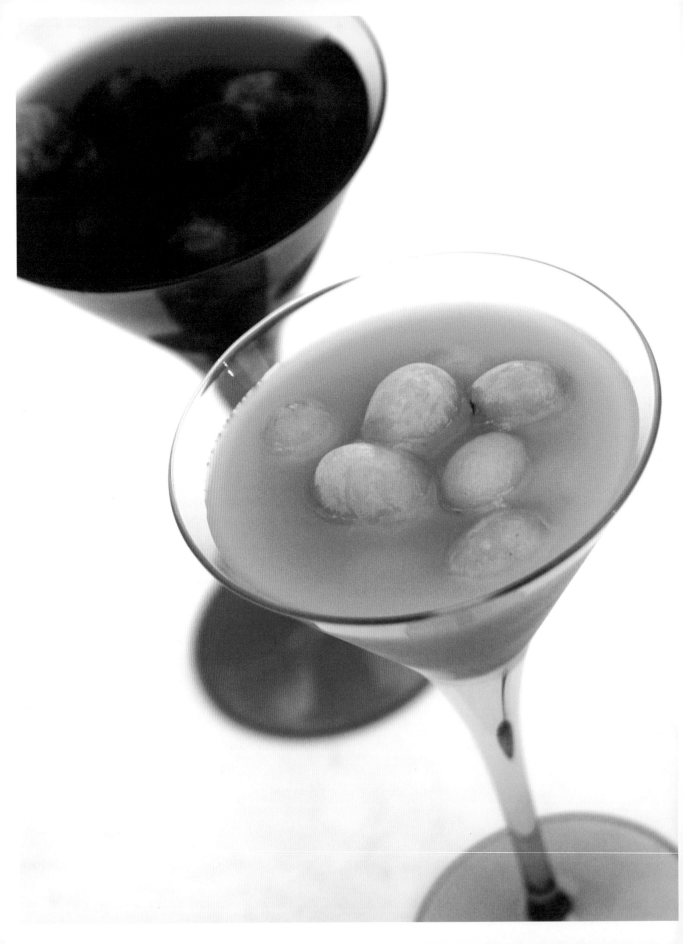

frozen grapes in juice

serves 4

nutrient	thumbs-up score
vitamin C	👍👍

Though not a nutritional heavyweight, this is great for tingling the tastebuds without filling you up too much. It acts a bit like an aperitif for something more nutritious.

24–30 large green & red seedless grapes
500ml chilled juice

Wash the grapes then arrange in a single layer to freeze overnight. (Plastic takeaway containers serve well for this task). When ready simply fill glasses with the grapes, pour the juice over and serve.

Each portion provides 0g protein and 75kcals

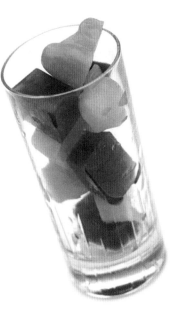

fruit juice ice cubes in yoghurt

serves 4

This is such a simple and delightful way to start the day. The juice cubes melt slowly so for a sore mouth or dry, delicate throat this drink is heaven and a great source of vitamin C.

500ml fruit juice or purée, (pineapple, mango, orange and cranberry)
a pinch of sugar, (if preparing purée it may need a touch of sweetness)
500ml yoghurt

Freeze the juice or purée in ice cube trays overnight.

To serve, place yoghurt in a blender with 125ml cold water and whip until frothy. Fill glasses with the juice cubes then pour in the yoghurt.

Each portion provides 8g protein and 210kcals

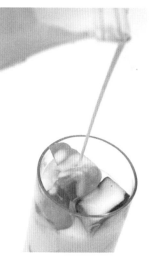

nutrient	thumbs-up score
vitamin C	>👍👍👍👍
vitamin A	👍
vitamin B12	👍
folate	👍
thiamin	👍
calcium	👍
phosphorus	👍

nutrient	thumbs-up score
vitamin C	👍👍👍
vitamin B6	👍
copper	👍

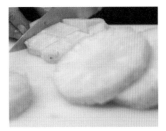

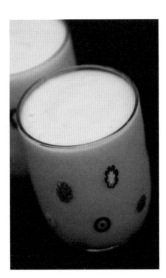

nutrient	thumbs-up score
vitamin C	>👍👍👍👍
vitamin B6	>👍👍👍👍
calcium	👍👍
fibre (non-starch polysaccaride)	👍👍
phosphorus	👍👍
iodine	👍👍
folate	👍👍
potassium	👍👍
magnesium	👍
iron	👍
copper	👍
thiamin	👍
riboflavin	👍
protein	👍

pineapple & ginger sherbet

serves 2 full portions or 4 light portions

This is another little tastebud zinger and is great when you need something soothing on the throat and don't have much appetite.

2 tbsp fresh peeled & grated ginger
½ medium pineapple, peeled, cored & chopped*
caster sugar to taste
handful of ice cubes

Place the ginger, pineapple and a teaspoon of sugar in a blender and purée until smooth. Add small amounts of water if the purée is too thick. Add further sugar if you prefer a sweeter drink.

Half fill a glass with ice shavings or cracked ice, fill the glass with purée, stir and serve immediately.

Each portion provides 1g protein and 120kcals

*see *the basics*, page 281

mango smoothie

serves 2 full or 4 light portions

Mango and yoghurt were made for each other. This is a lovely, fruity drink with bags of goodness.

100g yoghurt
250ml pineapple juice
1 slice pineapple, skin & eyes removed *
2 mangos, skin and stone removed
ice cubes

The method is the same as set out on page 28.

Each portion provides 9g protein and 320kcals

*see *the basics*, page 281

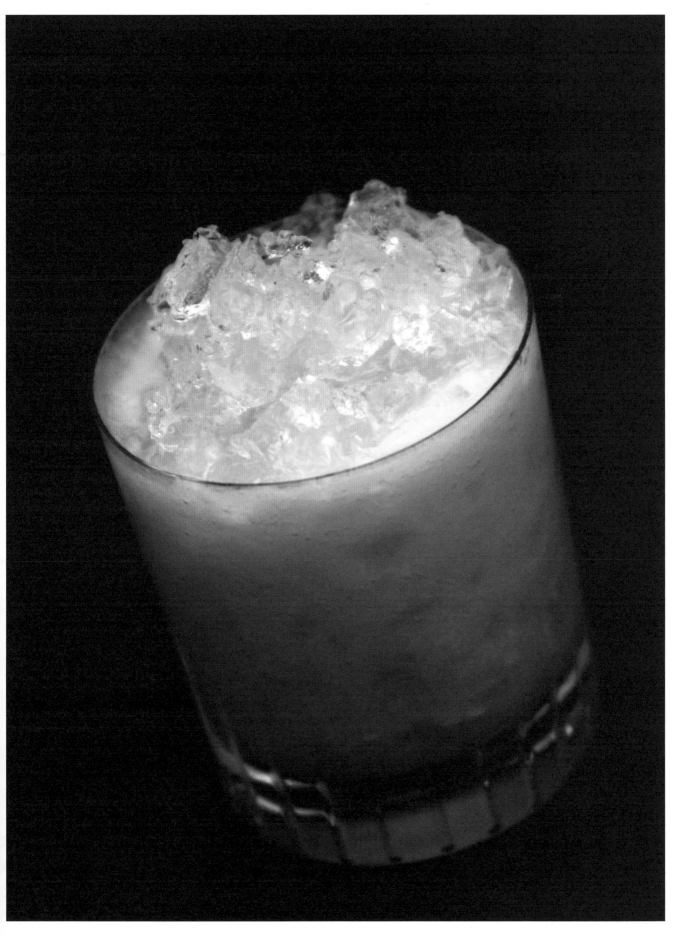

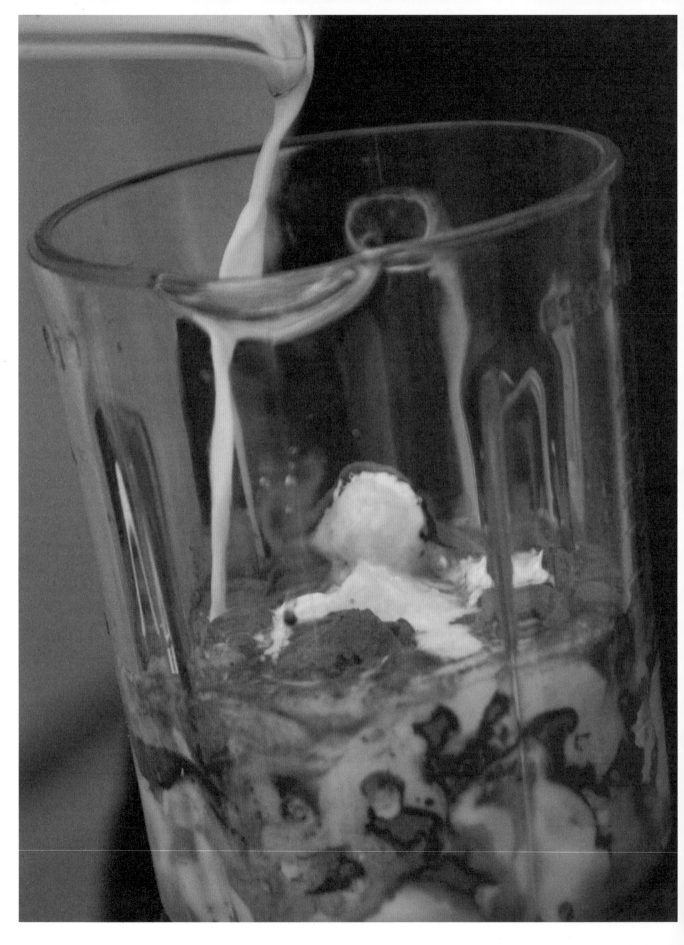

chocolate banana smoothie
serves 2 full or 4 light portions

Chocolate for breakfast is decadent. It'll start your day with a smile.

2-3 tbsp chocolate drink powder (or to taste)
1 banana
150ml milk
150g yoghurt
ice cubes, shaved or finely cracked

The method is the same as set out on page 28.

Each portion provides 8g protein and 190kcals

nutrient	thumbs-up score
iodine	👍👍👍
vitamin B12	👍👍
phosphorus	👍👍
vitamin B6	👍
vitamin C	👍
riboflavin	👍
calcium	👍
copper	👍

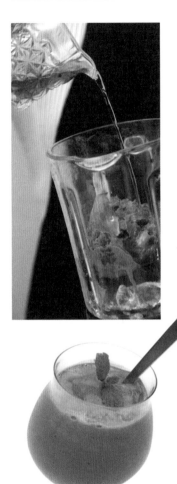

crème de menthe & chocolate frippery
serves 2 full portions

Yumola! Ok maybe it's not exactly a breakfast drink but sometimes you have to say, 'Life is uncertain, eat dessert first!'

100g frozen chocolate yoghurt
25-50ml crème de menthe, or 1 tbsp mint extract
splash of milk
chocolate shavings
sprig of fresh mint

Scoop the frozen yoghurt into a blender. Add the crème de menthe and splash of milk and whiz until thick and smooth. Add more milk if too thick and a bit of ice if too thin. Dust with chocolate shavings and garnish with mint.

Each portion provides 2g protein and 170kcals

nutrient	thumbs-up score
vitamin B12	👍

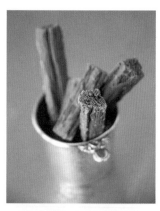

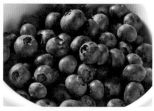

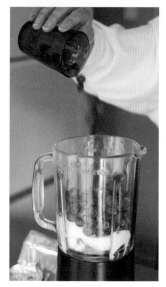

blueberry & yoghurt whippie
serves 2 full portions

There is something serenely appealing about the colour and texture of this little number and I can't decide whether it's a breakfast or pudding! Having said that, blueberries and chocolate, mmm.

100g frozen yoghurt
250ml blueberries, frozen (reserve a few for garnish)
splash of milk
1 chocolate flake per serving

Place the frozen blueberries and yoghurt in a blender and whiz until smooth. If you want a creamier drink, add a bit of milk. If you prefer a frozen parfait spoon the mixture into a glass and place back in the freezer for 20 minutes or add some ice while blending. Garnish with fresh blueberries and chocolate flake.

Each portion provides 4g protein and 260kcals

nutrient	thumbs-up score
vitamin B6	>👍👍👍👍
vitamin B12	👍👍
vitamin C	👍👍
phosphorus	👍

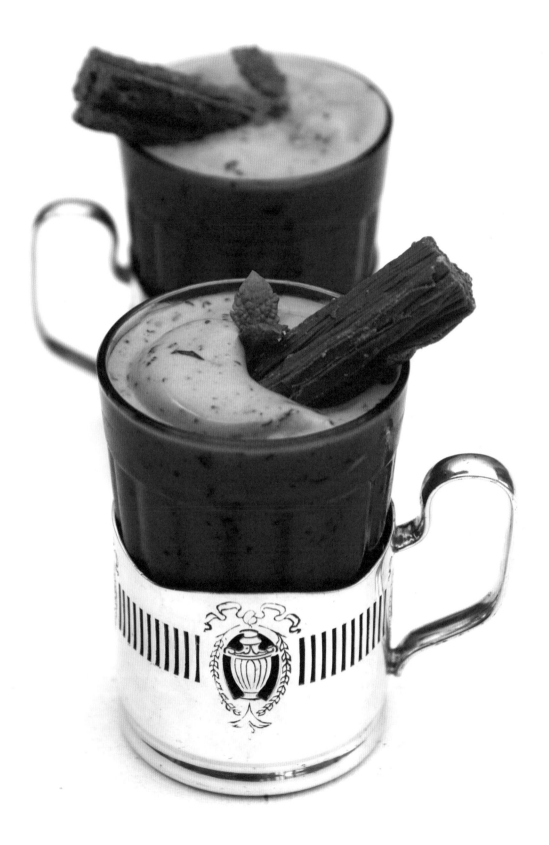

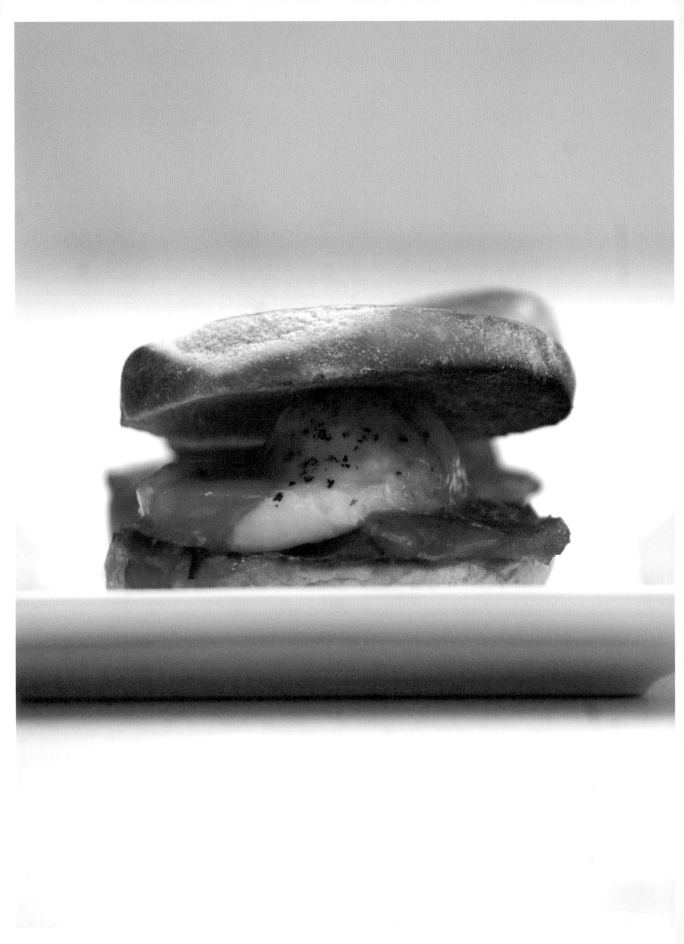

bacon & egger

serves 1

This is breakfast to go loved the world over and there is nothing better than starting a busy day with something to keep you going. Why not be your own drive-thru.

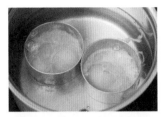

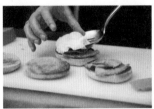

1 english muffin, halved and toasted
1 fresh, free-range egg
1 slice cheddar cheese
1 piece back bacon, fat removed
small amount of butter
salt & pepper

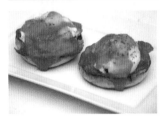

Fry the bacon in a small pan. Poach the egg* or as an alternative, beat the egg enough to break and mix the yolk with the white, add a bit of seasoning, pour into a plastic cup and pop into a microwave for 1 minute or until cooked through.

Toast and butter the muffin then build your sandwich. As a final touch, pop the sandwich back into the microwave for 10 seconds to gently melt the cheese. Wrap it in some parchment and away you go, day started!

Each portion provides 32g protein and 560kcals

*see *the basics*, page 282

nutrient	thumbs-up score
vitamin B12	>👍👍👍👍
sodium	👍👍👍👍
chloride	👍👍👍👍
calcium	👍👍👍
phosphorus	👍👍👍
vitamin A (total retinol equivalents)	👍👍
vitamin B6	👍👍
riboflavin	👍👍
thiamin	👍👍
protein	👍👍
folate	👍
niacin	👍
iodine	👍
iron	👍
selenium	👍
zinc	👍

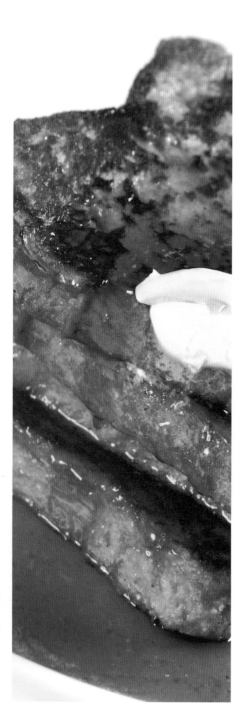

old-fashioned french toast
serves 4

Though not a nutritional giant french toast is comfort food at its best and is a great part of a full breakfast. Add your favourite fresh berries for added nutrition and flavour.

8 slices day old white bread

4 eggs

250ml milk

½ tsp cinnamon

butter

maple syrup to serve

Mix eggs, milk and cinnamon in a shallow dish.

Melt a knob of butter in a medium hot pan taking care not to burn. Next dip a bread slice on both sides so it is wet but not soggy. Fry in the pan to golden on both sides then remove and keep warm. Repeat with the rest of the slices.

Serve with maple syrup and a dollop of butter.

Each portion provides 5g protein and 210kcals

nutrient	thumbs-up score
sodium	👍
chloride	👍
selenium	👍

perfect poached eggs with beans on toast
serves 4, 1 egg per serving

This breakfast simply can't be improved on. I've had many a chemo suite conversation about the best method of poaching an egg. I've included a few here but use the method you like best.

4 fresh, free range eggs
1 tin baked beans
8 bacon rashers, fried
4 slices toast
lashings of butter

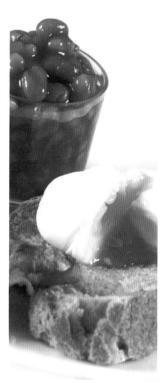

There are many methods for poaching eggs*. One sure-fire method is to lay a flat plate on the bottom of a pan to prevent the eggs from sticking. Add enough water for a cracked egg to be submerged in and heat to 80°C. Gently crack and drop in the egg. Cook for a couple minutes until the white is cooked and the yolk is hot but still soft. Remove with a slotted spoon and remove excess moisture on kitchen roll. Serve hot with toast, rashers of bacon and warmed beans.

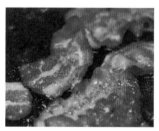

For alternative methods of poaching, there are silicon moulds that you can drop the egg into and place in simmering water or my favourite is to take a coffee mug and using cling film make a pocket in the mug. Crack the egg into the pocket then twist the top tightly shut. Float the film-wrapped egg in 80°C water for a few minutes, remove from water, unwrap and serve.

Each portion provides 9g protein and 215kcals

*see *the basics*, page 282

nutrient	thumbs-up score
vitamin B12	>👍👍👍👍
vitamin A total retinol equivalents)	👍
phosphorus	👍
selenium	👍

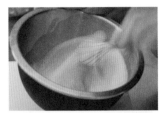

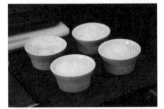

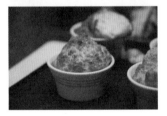

cheese soufflé

serves 4 as a starter, 2 as a main

Soufflés are such a lovely way to serve eggs which are often one of the few foods that one can tolerate when undergoing treatment.

1 15 cm soufflé dish or 4 ramekins

melted butter to grease dishes

fine white bread crumbs

40g butter

30g plain flour

½ tsp english mustard powder

drop of sriracha or pinch of cayenne

300ml milk, warmed

80g cheese, grated (gruyere, parmesan, roquefort or cheddar)

4 large eggs, separated

salt & pepper

Preheat oven to 200°Cf and place a baking tray higher than centre.

Make sure your dish or ramekins are very clean and dry, then brush with melted butter and very lightly dust with bread crumbs.

Next, in a heavy saucepan, melt the butter on low heat, stir in the flour then add the mustard and sriracha and let cook for just one minute. (If using roquefort or blue cheese forgo the mustard). Gradually add the milk until the mixture is smooth and comes to the boil. Stir constantly. Allow to boil for 2 minutes. The mixture should get quite thick and leave the sides of the pan.

Remove from the heat and stir in the cheese and egg yolks. Season to taste. It should be thick but able to pour.

In a separate, clean and dry bowl, whisk the egg whites until just stiff then add a spoonful to the cheese mixture. Gently fold in the remainder and pour into the soufflé dish or ramekins to ¾ full.

Bake for approximately 20-30 minutes for the large dish and 8-10 minutes for the ramekins. Do not open the oven door until ¾ through the baking time. To check for readiness give the dish a little push. If the soufflé wobbles, cook for about 5 minutes more for large and 1 for small. Serve immediately.

Each portion provides 9g protein and 260kcals

nutrient	thumbs-up score
vitamin B12	👍👍👍
potassium	👍
vitamin A (total retinol equivalents)	👍
iodine	👍
phosphorus	👍
sodium	👍
chloride	👍

(our analysis has been done as 4 individual ramekins)

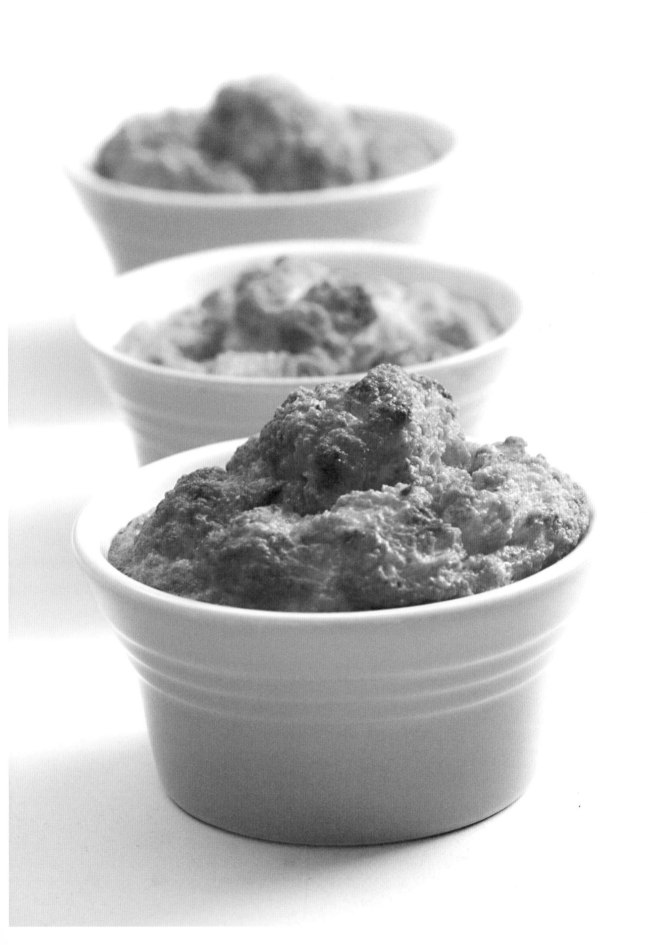

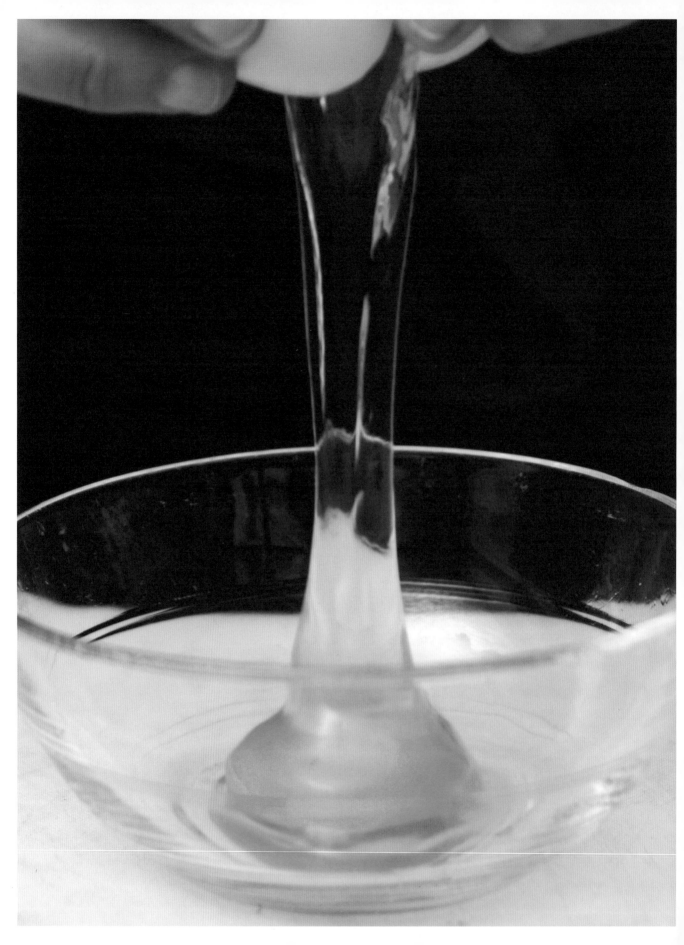

savoury egg cupcakes
serves 6, 2 cupcakes per person

These little bundles of happiness are a super fast way to prepare a light and nutritious meal and a great way to use leftovers. Serve with a mesclun* salad and blue cheese dressing† for a light lunch.

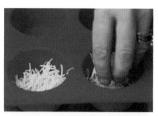

8 large, free-range eggs

4 chipolatas, bacon or ham

100g emmenthal cheese, or cheddar, finely grated

300ml sour cream

300ml milk

1 tsp savoury, or mixed herbs

salt & pepper

small knob of butter

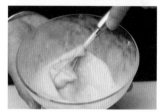

For this dish I use silicon cupcake moulds

Preheat oven to 160°Cf.

Bake the chipolatas until well cooked and allow to rest on paper towel to absorb excess fat. When rested, cut into sufficient slices to create a bottom layer for 12 cupcakes. Sprinkle some grated cheese onto the chipolatas.

Crack eggs into a bowl and using a fork beat in sour cream, milk and savoury until smooth. Be careful not to add too much air. Add a bit of seasoning.

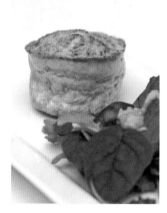

If using silicon moulds, place them on a baking tray, lightly butter then pour the egg mixture into the moulds to ¾ full. Place in central position in oven and allow to bake until fully cooked, about 15-20 minutes. When finished they should be well risen and springy but not turning colour. Serve immediately.

Each portion provides 10g protein and 270kcals

*see *the basics*, page 284

†see *the basics*, page 284

nutrient	thumbs-up score
vitamin B12	👍👍👍
vitamin A (total retinol equivalents)	👍👍
calcium	👍👍
phosphorus	👍👍
sodium	👍👍
chloride	👍👍
riboflavin	👍
copper	👍
protein	👍

waffles

serves 4

These waffles are light, fluffy and crunchy in one. They're best right off the grittle and reheat well. This is breakfast that craves good company.

160g flour
4 tsp baking powder
½ tsp salt
2 tsp sugar
100g butter, melted
400ml milk
2 eggs, separated
2-3 extra knobs of butter for cooking

your choice of toppings for serving

butter & maple syrup
crème fraiche & blackberries
strawberries & cream
nutella & bananas

You will need a waffle iron to prepare this dish.

In a dry, clean bowl, sift together the dry ingredients, beat in the egg yolks then whisk in the milk and melted butter. Next beat the egg whites until fairly stiff and fold them into the batter.

Wam a waffle iron to medium heat and brush with butter then spoon on mixture. Cook until lightly golden then flip and cook the same on the other side.

Keep waffles warm and serve with favourite toppings.

**Each portion provides 5g protein and 480kcals
(3 strawberries and 25ml double cream used for analysis)**

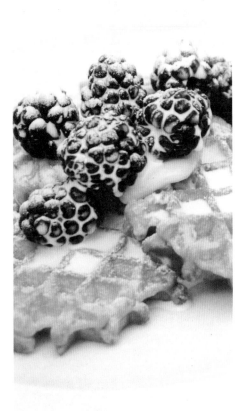

nutrient	thumbs-up score
vitamin A (total retinol equivalents)	👍👍👍👍
vitamin B12	👍👍👍👍
phosphorus	👍👍👍👍
vitamin C	👍👍👍
sodium	👍👍👍
riboflavin	👍
iodine	👍
calcium	👍
chloride	👍

crèpes
serves 6, 2 crèpes per serving

I always associate crèpes with special occasions and times to be savoured and enjoyed. Frankly, if you'd rather spend more time enjoying and less time with a crèpe pan, buy them ready made.

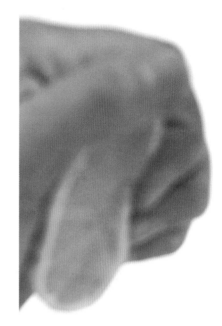

200g plain flour
1 tsp sugar
½ tsp salt
zest of 1 orange
450ml milk
2 eggs
a couple knobs of butter for cooking

filling of choice
cream cheese & sultanas
sugar & lemon curd (or lemon juice)
yoghurt & berries
butter & raspberry jam

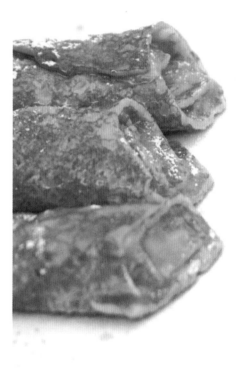

Sift together flour, sugar and salt then mix in orange zest then make a well in the middle. In a separate bowl, beat together the milk and eggs and pour this into the well. Beat mixture until smooth.

Next preheat a pan on medium heat. Using a piece of parchment, coat the pan with butter then pour in 50g of the batter and quickly tilt in a circular motion to evenly coat the pan with batter. Cook until lightly golden, about 2 minutes, then flip and do the same for the other side. Serve hot with your favourite filling.

Each portion provides 3g protein and 150kcals
(10g lemon curd and 4g icing sugar used for analysis)

nutrient	thumbs-up score
vitamin B12	👍👍
vitamin C	👍

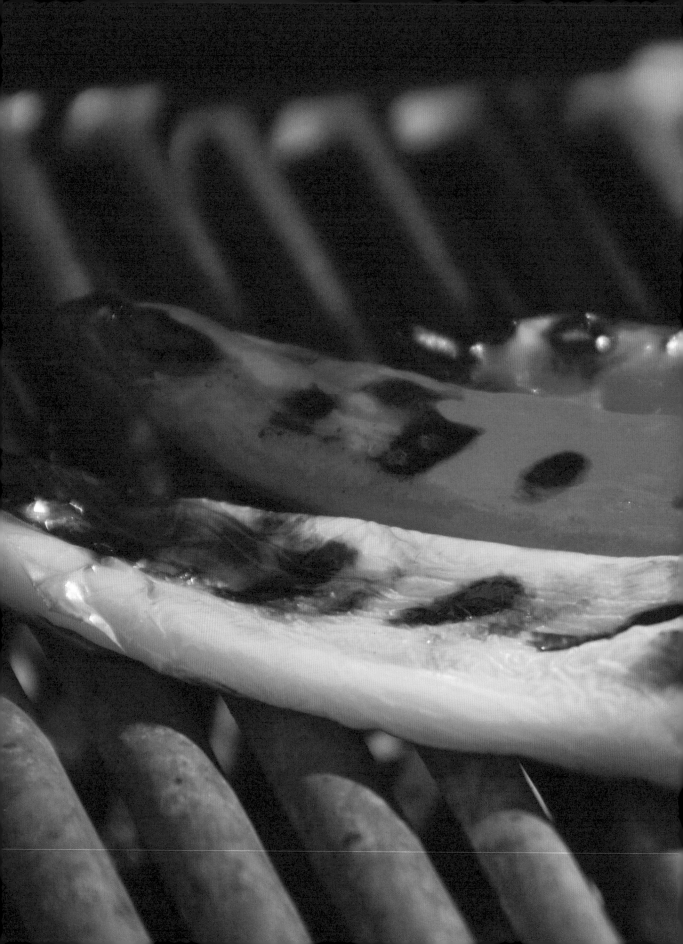

grazing

grazing

italian stuffed bread 53

goat's cheese & chestnut crumble tart 54

chicken liver parfait 57

cheese straws 58

hummus & pitta toasties 61

bbq salsa, guacamole & tortilla chips 62

smoked salmon & caviar blinis 64

marinated pepper & goat's cheese crostini 65

welsh rarebit 67

quails eggs with mushroom duxelle & hollandaise 68

wild mushroom tart 69

prawn avocado cocktail 71

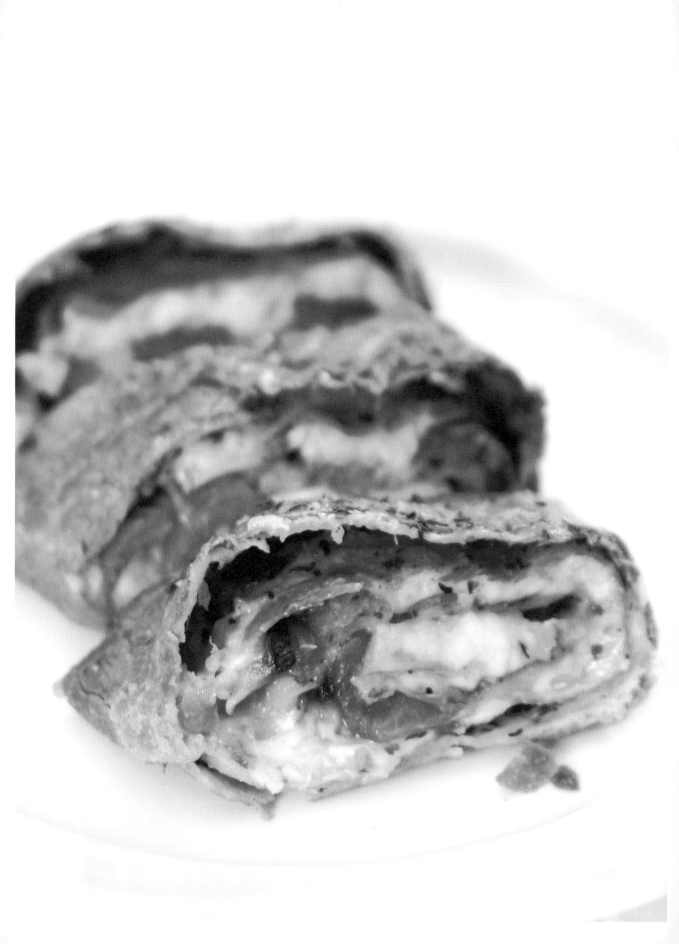

italian stuffed bread
1 loaf serves 4 as a starter or snack

This is one of your best friends for so many reasons. Tomatoes and mushrooms for a start. It's filled with good nutrition and crammed with flavour. It's so fast and simple.

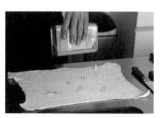

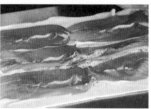

pre-made croissant dough or puff pastry*
olive oil
8-10 fine slices parma ham
8-10 fine slices mozzarella cheese
2 large tomatoes, finely sliced
6-8 white mushrooms, finely sliced
dried italian herbs
salt & pepper
1 egg, whisked

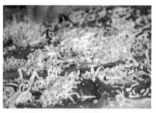

Preheat the oven to 170°Cf.

*There are two easy ways to prepare the dough. I prefer the croissant dough but puff pastry works as well. The pre-made croissant dough usually comes in a tube and is perforated into triangles. Remove the dough and make a large rectangle of dough by squidging together perforated edges. It does work.

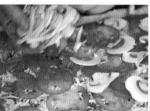

On a floured surface, roll out the dough into a rectangle the thickness of fine piecrust. Brush with a thin film of olive oil. Layer the ham, cheese, tomatoes and mushrooms. Sprinkle generously with herbs, salt and pepper. Roll up and tuck the ends under, brush all over with egg wash and bake for about 20 minutes until golden brown. Allow to set for about 5 minutes. Slice and serve warm.

Each portion provides 35g protein and 740kcals

nutrient	thumbs-up score
sodium	>👍👍👍👍
chloride	>👍👍👍👍
folate	👍👍👍👍
vitamin B6	👍👍👍
vitamin B12	👍👍👍
protein	👍👍👍
vitamin A (total retinol equivalents)	👍👍
calcium	👍👍
copper	👍👍
iron	👍👍
phosphorus	👍👍
vitamin C	👍
riboflavin	👍
thiamin	👍
fibre (as non-starch polysaccharide)	👍
magnesium	👍
zinc	👍

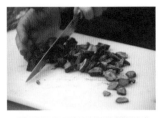

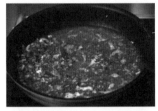

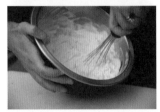

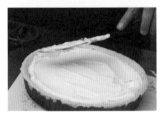

goat's cheese & chestnut crumble tart

yield 1 tart

This traditional tart is such a nice dish for lunch. So light and savoury. It's perfect with watercress & crispy shallot salad.

500g soft goat's cheese
100ml single cream
1 egg and 2 yolks
8 inch pastry case, blind-baked*
1 tbsp butter
1 clove garlic, crushed
200g chestnuts, peeled and finely chopped
200ml chicken stock
1 bay leaf

Preheat oven to 160°Cf.

Remove any skin from the cheese then beat with the cream and eggs until smooth. Pour into the blind-baked pastry case and bake for 20 minutes or until set. Set aside to cool.

For the crumble, warm the butter in a pan with the garlic and cook without colour. Add the chopped chestnuts, stock and bay leaf and simmer until the chestnuts are tender. Drain well and spread over paper towel to remove excess moisture. When cool sprinkle evenly over the surface of the tart.

Return to the oven to warm before serving.

Each portion provides 19g protein and 643kcals

*see *the basics*, page 284

nutrient	thumbs-up score
vitamin B6	👍👍👍👍
vitamin A total retinol equivalents)	👍👍👍
sodium	👍👍👍
chloride	👍👍👍
vitamin C	👍👍
iron	👍👍
folate	👍
thiamin	👍
calcium	👍
copper	👍
fibre (non-starch polysaccaride)	👍
magnesium	👍
phosphorus	👍
protein	👍
zinc	👍

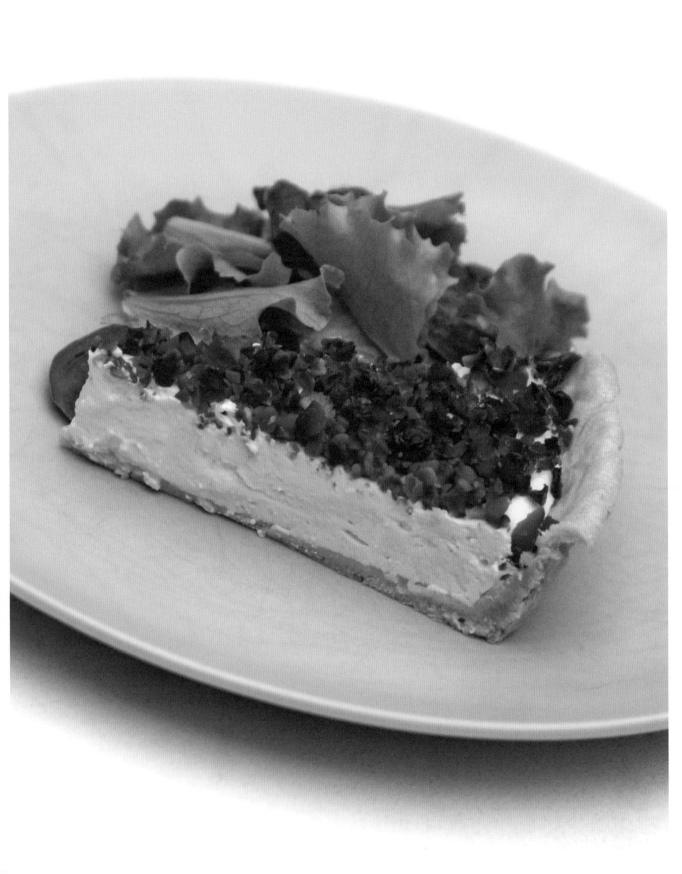

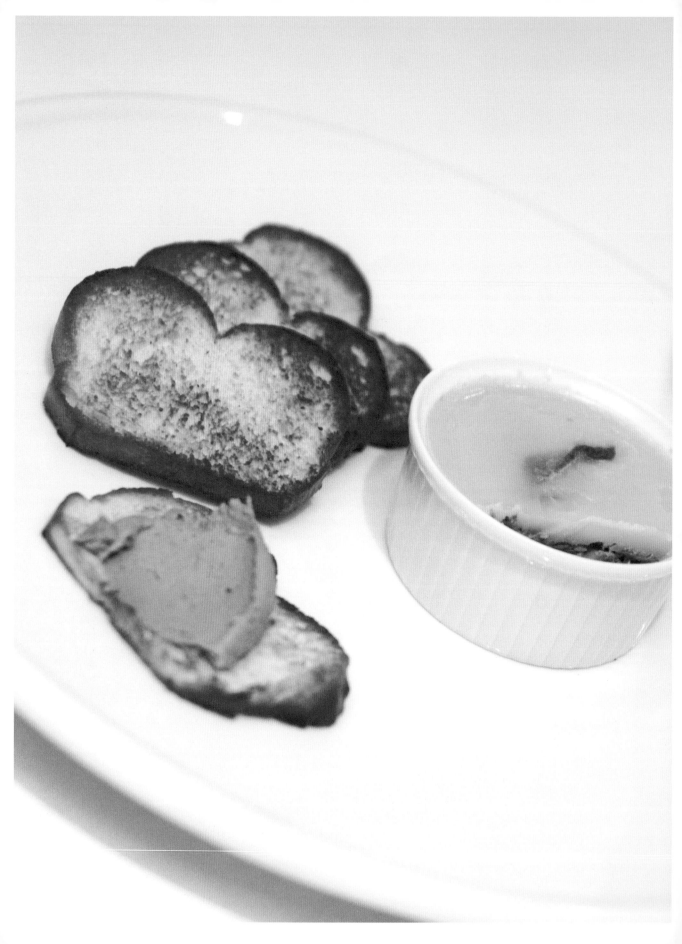

chicken liver parfait

serves 4

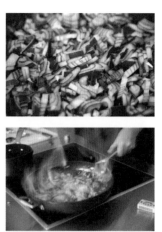

Chicken liver is one of the best sources of iron. It's a lovely hors d'oeuvre but it's pretty calorific. Go on, live a little!

500g butter
small bunch of fresh sage, leaves picked
olive oil
1 red onion, finely chopped
1 clove garlic, finely chopped
small bunch of fresh thyme
500g chicken livers, trimmed
salt & freshly ground black pepper
small wine glass of brandy
toasted brioche to serve

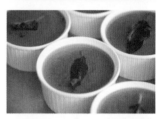

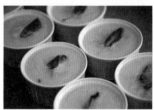

Start by clarifying 250g butter*. Keep on medium-high heat and add a sage leaf and continue to warm allowing the sage to infuse. When the leaf is crisp remove it and add the rest of the leaves to deep fry until crispy. Remove and drain on kitchen paper.

Next coat a pan with oil, and add the onion, garlic and thyme. Sauté for about 4 minutes until soft and starting to colour. Add a splash more oil and the chicken livers and lightly season. Cook on high heat for 4 minutes. The livers will plump up and you want them soft and pink inside. They become tough when overcooked.

Next warm the brandy then pour it onto the livers and flambé if you like. Allow to simmer for about 1 minute. Transfer the mixture into a food processor and purée until very smooth then add a knob of butter continuing to purée until the butter is fully melted.

Dice the remaining 250g of butter and add it piece by piece, with the food processor running. Adjust the seasoning bearing in mind that it will mellow as the mixture cools.

Finally, push through a sieve and pour the mixture into individual ramekins. When set, cover with remaining clarified butter and garnish with a crispy sage leaf. Place back in the fridge.

Each portion provides 24g protein and 1270kcals

*see *the basics*, page 280

nutrient	thumbs-up score
vitamin A (total retinol equivalents)	>👍👍👍👍
vitamin B6	>👍👍👍👍
vitamin B12	>👍👍👍👍
folate	>👍👍👍👍
riboflavin	>👍👍👍👍
iron	>👍👍👍👍
sodium	👍👍👍
chloride	👍👍👍
potassium	👍👍👍
vitamin C	👍👍
niacin	👍👍
thiamin	👍👍
copper	👍👍
protein	👍👍
zinc	👍👍
vitamin D	👍
calcium	👍

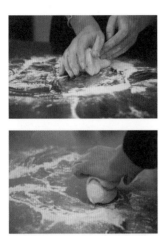

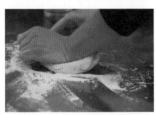

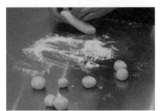

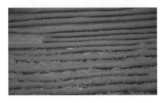

cheese straws
yields 12 large sticks

These are a fun little nibble and great to serve with pasta or soups.
If you want to add to their nutritional value use whole grain flour.

This is the same dough I use for pizza.

15g fresh yeast with a splash of warm water or 1½ tsp dried yeast
250g flour, type 00 hard durum wheat or strong bread
1 tsp salt
50ml olive oil
225g parmesan or emmenthal cheese, finely grated

Preheat oven to 180°Cf.

Sift the flour and salt into a large mixing bowl and make a well in the middle. Drizzle in the oil and add the yeast. Mix with a wooden spoon, adding splashes of water as required, to make a soft dough. Turn out onto a floured surface and knead for 10-12 minutes until smooth and elastic. Don't scrimp on kneading time!

Split the dough into 2 balls and place in a lightly oiled bowl, giving each ball a light coating of oil. Cover and leave in a warm place for about 1½ hours.

Flatten out the dough and knead again on a lightly floured surface for 2-3 minutes. At this stage you can wrap the dough and freeze for future use.

Roll out dough into 12 inch snakes. Brush lightly with olive oil and sprinkle with salt and finely grated parmesan or emmenthal cheese. Bake until golden and crisp.

Each portion provides 19g protein and 300kcals

nutrient	thumbs-up score
vitamin B12	👍👍👍👍
calcium	👍👍👍
chloride	👍👍
phosphorus	👍👍
vitamin A (total retinol equivalents)	👍
folate	👍
copper	👍
iodine	👍
protein	👍
sodium	👍
zinc	👍

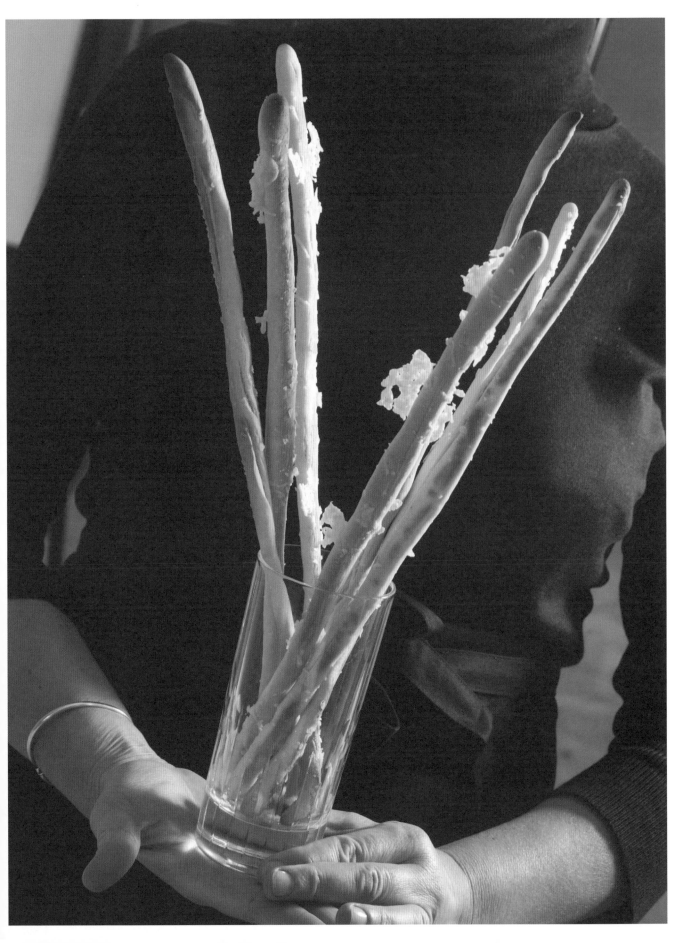

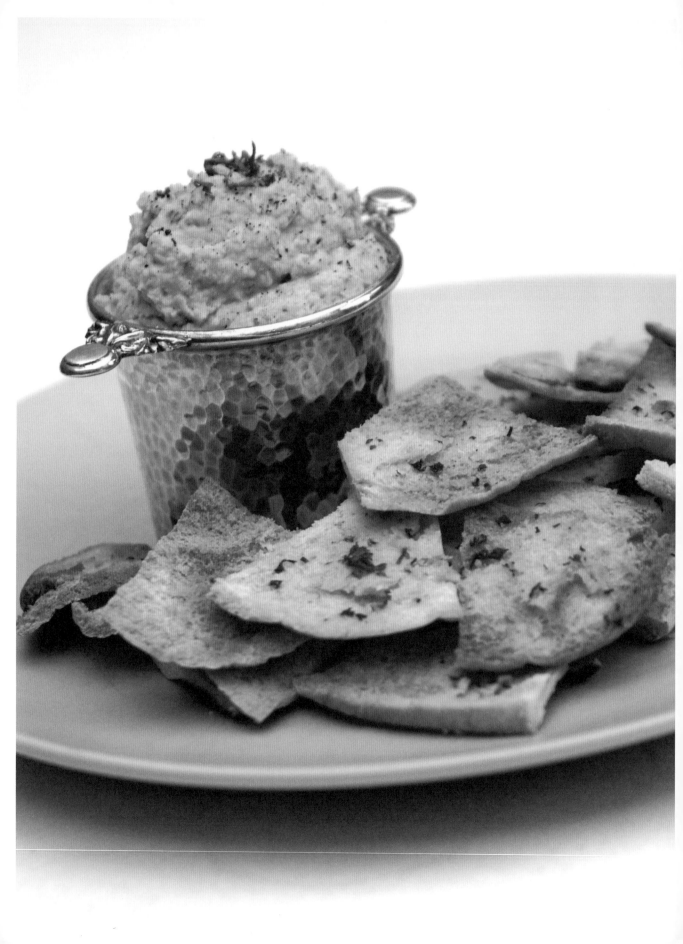

hummus & pitta toasties
serves 6

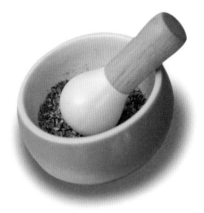

*This snack is a great source of minerals, especially iron. The flavour is
simply bigger and better when made fresh.*

for the hummus
424g chickpeas, 1 tin drained and rinsed
50g tahini
juice of 1 lemon
2 cloves garlic, puréed
½ tsp ground cumin
½ tsp salt
1 small bunch parsley, finely chopped
1 tsp sesame oil
1 tbsp olive oil

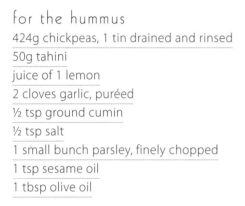

for the pitta toasties
6-8 rounds pitta bread
175g butter
2 tbsp parsley, finely chopped
1 tbsp chives, finely chopped
1 clove garlic, puréed
1 tsp lemon juice
salt & pepper

Place the chickpeas, tahini, lemon juice, garlic, cumin and salt in a
blender. Mix until smooth, adding drops of water until creamy.

Place the mixture in a bowl and stir in the parsley and oils. Chill for
at least 30 minutes and garnish with paprika to serve.

Next whip the butter, parsley, chives, garlic and lemon juice into a
smooth paste. Roll into cling film and refrigerate until ready to use.

Preheat oven to 180°Cf.

Open the pitta rounds and cut into bite-sized pieces and place on
a baking tray. Melt butter and lightly brush the pitta pieces then
place in the oven until just turning golden. Serve warm.

Each portion provides 14g protein and 550kcals

nutrient	thumbs-up score
vitamin A total retinol equivalents)	👍👍👍
sodium	👍👍👍
chloride	👍👍👍
vitamin C	👍👍
iron	👍👍
folate	👍
thiamin	👍
calcium	👍
copper	👍
fibre (non-starch polysaccharide)	👍
magnesium	👍
phosphorus	👍
protein	👍
zinc	👍

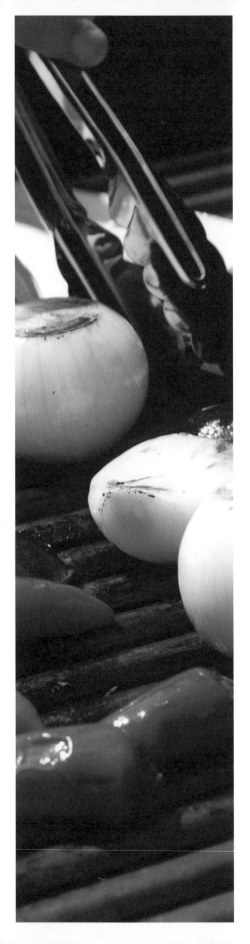

bbq salsa, guacamole & tortilla chips

yields approximately 2 cups of each, a snack for 4-6 people

This is great grazing food and an easy way to digest vegetables. Add more lime to the guacamole for a stronger flavour. A small amount delivers a lot of vitamins and minerals.

salsa

olive oil

2 large onions, peeled

1 aubergine, thickly sliced

2 courgette, thickly sliced

3 jalapeno peppers

3 bell peppers

4 large italian tomatoes

1 whole bulb garlic

small bunch coriander, chopped

salt & pepper

Preheat a bbq grill until very hot, around 400°C.

Coat the vegetables and garlic with olive oil then grill until lightly charred. Start with the onions as they take the longest. Leave the tomatoes until last. Remove from the grill.

When the peppers are well charred on the outside, sweat them in a sealed container or plastic bag. When cool enough to handle, remove the skins and seeds.

Squeeze the garlic flesh out of the husks and place in a food processor with the grilled vegetables. Blend gently until evenly mixed but not puréed. Add coriander and season to taste. Serve with tortilla chips.

guacamole

3 ripe medium size avocados, peeled and stoned

1 large italian tomato, chopped and seeds removed

juice of 1 lime

small bunch coriander, chopped

¼ cup crème fraiche

salt & pepper

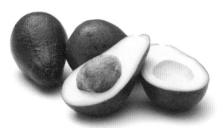

Place the avocado meat in a bowl and coarsely mash. Fold in the remaining ingredients. If preparing in advance, store in an airtight container. Serve with tortilla chips.

tortilla chips

Preheat oven to grill.

Cut soft flour tortillas into bite-sized triangles, place on a baking sheet and grill until just turning golden.

Each portion provides 12g protein and 595kcals

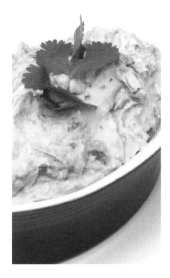

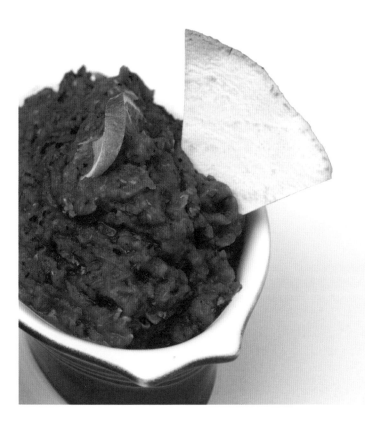

nutrient	thumbs-up score
vitamin B6	>👍👍👍
vitamin C	>👍👍👍
vitamin A (total retinol equivalents	👍👍👍
fibre (as a non-starch polysaccaride)	👍👍👍
folate	👍👍👍
thiamin	👍👍
phosphorus	👍👍
potassium	👍👍
sodium	👍👍
chloride	👍👍
niacin	👍
riboflavin	👍
calcium	👍
copper	👍
iron	👍
magnesium	👍
protein	👍

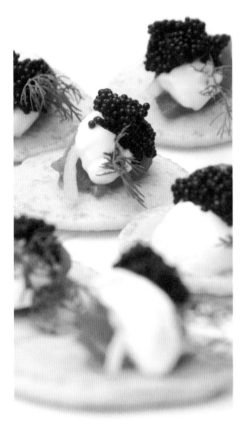

smoked salmon & caviar blinis
serves 4-6

The caviar is a real sensation, It's strong and has lots of texture both for the eyes and in the mouth. This is definitely a best friend for strength of flavour and combination of textures.

8-10 sheets filo pastry, or substitute with store bought blinis
melted butter
1 egg
fine breadcrumbs
smoked alaska wild salmon, cut into 10g strips
1 jar lumpfish caviar
sour cream
lemon rind, cut into fine julienne
fresh dill sprigs

Preheat oven to 200°Cf.

To prepare the filo squares, place a layer on a baking sheet then lightly brush with melted butter and egg wash. Then sprinkle with fine breadcrumbs. Place another layer of pastry on top and repeat with the butter, eggwash and crumbs until you have 8-10 layers. Cut into 1½ -2 inch squares then bake until golden brown. Remove from oven and allow to cool.

Twist a strip of salmon onto a filo square then fill with soured cream. Top with caviar and garnish with lemon rind and dill. Easy peasy!

**Each portion provides 19g protein and 560kcals
(30g protein and 750kcals with blinis)**

nutrient	thumbs-up score
vitamin B12	>👍👍👍👍
sodium	>👍👍👍👍
chloride	>👍👍👍👍
phosphorus	>👍👍👍👍
vitamin A total retinol equivalents)	👍👍👍
vitamin B6	👍👍👍
riboflavin	👍👍
calcium	👍👍
protein	👍👍
vitamin D	👍
thiamin	👍
iron	👍
potassium	👍
selenium	👍
zinc	👍

marinated pepper & goat's cheese crostini

yields approximately 30 pieces

The power of the pepper! These are great little bites that burst with flavour. The marinated peppers will last for a couple weeks if refrigerated in a sealed container.

3 red peppers

olive oil

garlic, crushed

fresh herbs, finely chopped

baguette, sliced and toasted

soft goat's cheese

nutrient	thumbs-up score
sodium	>👍👍👍👍
chloride	>👍👍👍👍
folate	👍👍👍👍
vitamin B6	👍👍👍
vitamin B12	👍👍👍
protein	👍👍👍
vitamin A (total retinol equivalents)	👍👍
calcium	👍👍
copper	👍👍
iron	👍👍
vitamin C	👍
riboflavin	👍
thiamin	👍
fibre (as non-starch polysaccharide)	👍
magnesium	👍
zinc	👍

Coat the peppers lightly with olive oil and grill until the skin is charred and blistered. Put in a plastic bag and leave to sweat. When cool, peel and soak in olive oil infused with garlic and a few herbs. To serve, slice finely and pile on toasted baguette spread with soft goat's cheese.

Each portion provides 12g protein and 290kcals

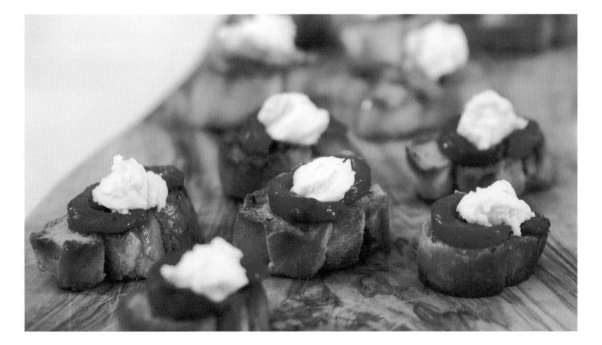

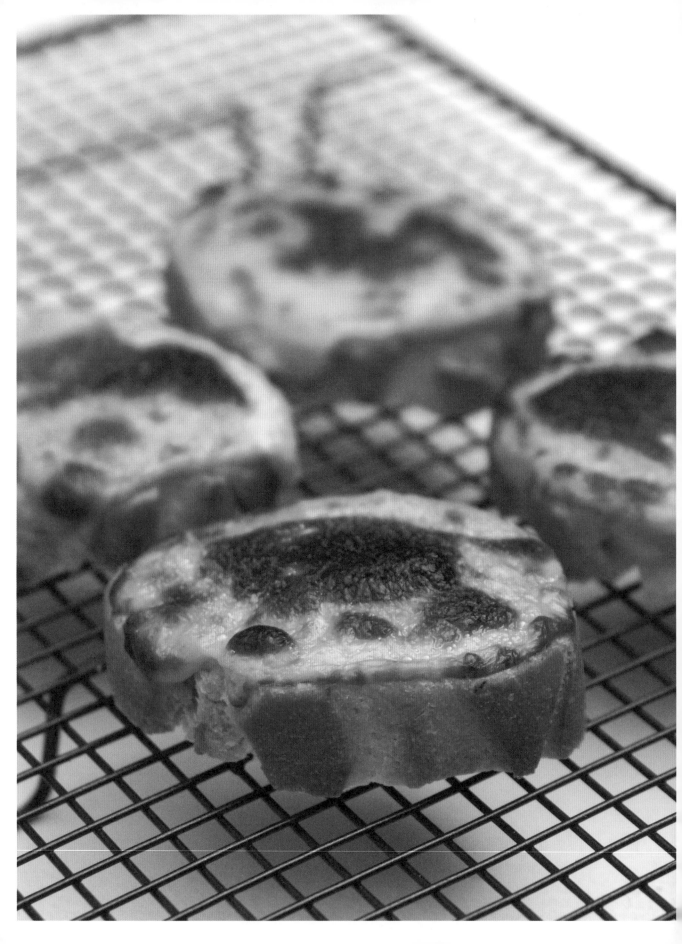

welsh rarebit

serves 8

Welsh rarebit has so much going for it. It's comforting, quick and packed with goodness. The worcestershire sauce, mustard and ale strengthen the flavour and might help cut through plastic and metal mouth.

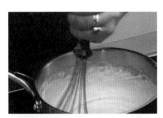

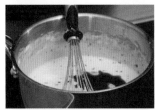

125ml milk
1 tbsp flour
400g sharp cheddar, grated
handful of fresh white breadcrumbs
1 heaped tsp english mustard powder
1 tbsp worcestershire sauce
120ml ale or cider
1 egg plus 1 yolk
crusty french bread slices, toasted

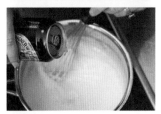

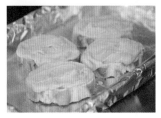

Heat the milk in a pan, whisk in flour and bring to the boil until slightly thickened. Reduce heat and add the grated cheese. Stir until melted, and then add the breadcrumbs, mustard, worcestershire sauce and ale. Continue to stir on low heat until the mixture starts to leave the side of the pan. Remove the heat and leave to cool slightly.

Next whisk in the egg and egg yolk until light and fluffy. Season to taste. Spread onto toast and grill until golden. Serve with watercress and a vinaigrette.*

One portion provides 46g protein and 1008kcals when served with 1 french stick and 20g portions of watercress with vinaigrette.

This mixture can be stored in the fridge for up to five days. Allow it to cool then seal in an airtight container. It will form a block that can be sliced. Try melting some on baked portobello mushrooms.

*see *the basics*, page 282

nutrient	thumbs-up score
vitamin B12	>👍👍👍👍
calcium	>👍👍👍👍
phosphorus	>👍👍👍👍
sodium	>👍👍👍👍
chloride	>👍👍👍👍
protein	👍👍👍👍
vitamin A (total retinol equivalents)	👍👍👍
zinc	👍👍👍
vitamin B6	👍👍
folate	👍👍
iodine	👍👍
riboflavin	👍👍
thiamin	👍
copper	👍
fibre (as non-starch polysaccharide)	👍
magnesium	👍
selenium	👍

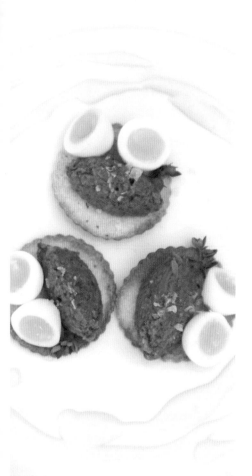

quails eggs with mushroom duxelle & hollandaise

serves 4

This is a medal winner for flavour and texture. It's a bit fiddly to prepare but so worth it. Most of it can be done well in advance.

8 quails eggs
5ml white wine vinegar
4 slices day old bread

mushroom duxelle
This recipe is on page 164

melba toast
Remove the crusts from the bread slices then roll thin with a rolling pin. Cut into rounds with a scone cutter and place on a baking sheet. Toast under the grill until lightly golden brown on both sides

to poach the quails eggs
Pour 2 inches of water into a pan and heat to the point where bubbles are formed on the bottom of the pan but the water isn't boiling. Stir in the vinegar. When ready to place the eggs in, give the water a gentle swirl.

To crack the eggs, gently pierce with the tip of a knife then very gently open taking care not to break the yolk. Place in the hot water for no more 1-1½ minutes then remove with a slotted spoon and drain on kitchen paper.

If you prefer, soft boil the eggs in boiling water for 1½ -2 minutes then plunge immediately into cold water to stop the cooking process. Peel and slice.

to assemble
Place a small quenelle of duxelle on the toast then stack with the egg and drizzle with hollandaise*.

Each portion provides 12g protein and 780kcals

*see *the basics*, page 281

nutrient	thumbs-up score
vitamin A (total retinol equivalents)	>👍👍👍👍
sodium	👍👍👍👍
chloride	👍👍👍👍
vitamin B12	👍👍👍
riboflavin	👍👍
copper	👍👍
phosphorus	👍👍
vitamin B6	👍
thiamin	👍
calcium	👍
iodine	👍
iron	👍
protein	👍

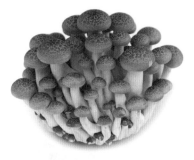

wild mushroom tart
yields 1 tart

Mushrooms, garlic, onion, eggs and three sources of calcium make this a sure-fire winner. Super for breakfast or lunch with a green salad.

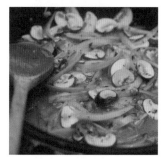

1 savoury pastry case (ready made is fine), blind-baked*

1 medium onion, sliced into fine rings

2 cups wild mushrooms

100ml olive oil

1 clove garlic, crushed

100ml white wine

3 eggs

100ml crème fraiche

50ml milk

herbs de provençe

1 cup gruyere cheese, grated

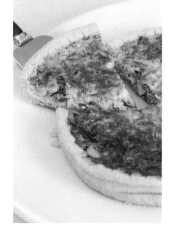

Preheat oven to 170°Cf.

Fry the onion in a little oil on a low heat until caramelised. In a separate pan, fry the mushrooms, oil, garlic and wine until the liquid has evaporated. Add the onions, stir to combine then spread evenly inside the pastry case.

Beat together the eggs, crème fraiche, milk and herbs. Stir in the grated cheese and pour over the vegetables. Place on a baking tray and bake for about 30 minutes until cooked through and lightly golden brown. Serve hot or cold.

Each portion provides 15g protein and 760kcals

*see *the basics*, page 280

nutrient	thumbs-up score
vitamin B6	>👍👍👍
vitamin B12	>👍👍👍
vitamin A (total retinol equivalents)	👍👍
phosphorus	👍👍
vitamin D	👍
riboflavin	👍
calcium	👍
copper	👍
iodine	👍
iron	👍
protein	👍
sodium	👍
chloride	👍

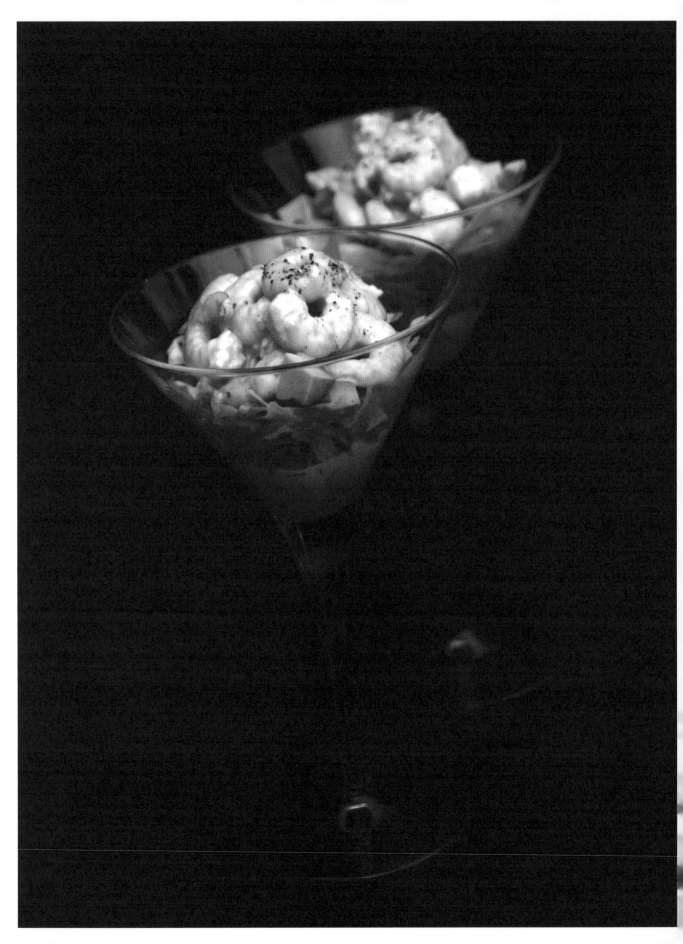

prawn avocado cocktail

serves 4

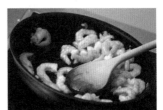

This classic has seen somewhat of a revival recently. It's no wonder, for simplicity, flavour and texture it's hard to beat. The Mary Rose sauce has a bit of an extra kick and be generous with it.

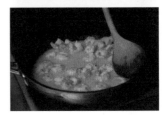

250ml prawns, peeled, deveined and cooked
2 ripe avocados
iceburg lettuce, very finely shredded
freshly cracked black pepper

mary rose sauce

4 tbsp mayonnaise
2 tsp ketchup
1 tsp horseradish, finely grated
juice & zest of 1 lime
dash of tabasco sauce
dash of worcestershire sauce
20ml vodka, (the extra kick)

To make the sauce stir all ingredients excluding the prawns, avocado and lettuce in a bowl. Add the prawns and coat with the sauce. Place in the fridge until ready to serve.

Halve the avocados and remove the stone and peel. Dice into bite-sized chunks. To serve arrange the avocado and prawns on a small bed of shredded lettuce. Add a good turn of fresh black pepper.

Each portion provides 16g protein and 430kcals

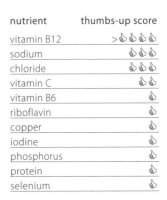

nutrient	thumbs-up score
vitamin B12	>👍👍👍👍
sodium	👍👍👍
chloride	👍👍👍
vitamin C	👍👍
vitamin B6	👍
riboflavin	👍
copper	👍
iodine	👍
phosphorus	👍
protein	👍
selenium	👍

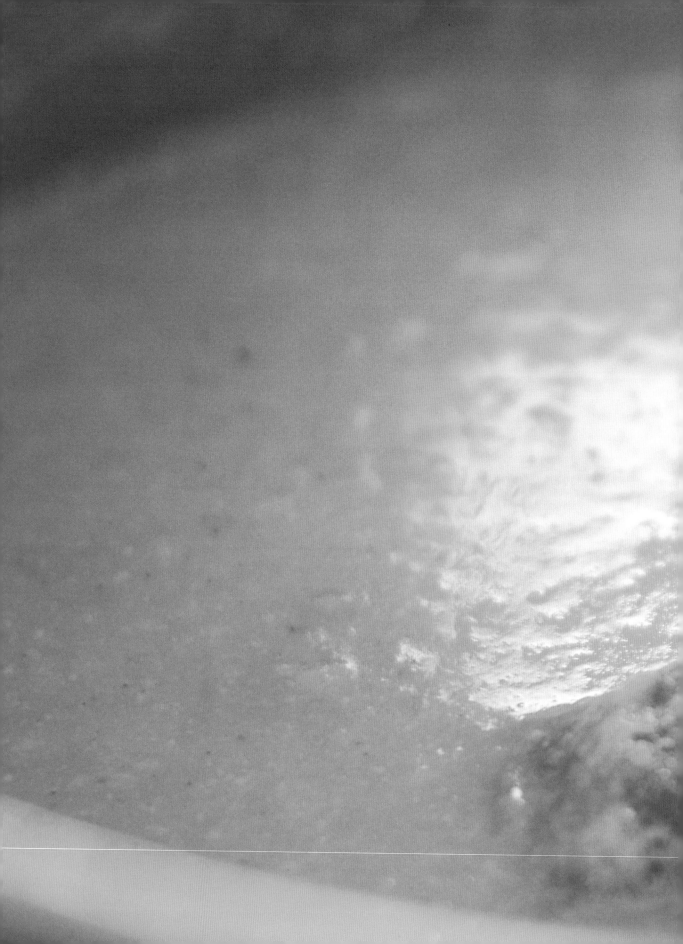

soups

soups

chestnut   77

prawn & ginger   78

creamy watercress   81

partridge cock-a-leekie   82

potato & leek pottage   83

sage, sweetcorn & onion chowder   85

white bean, sausage & kale   86

spicy pumpkin   89

nova scotia clam chowder   90

rich russian borscht   93

cream of cauliflower & cumin   94

cream of mushroom   95

tuscan bean   96

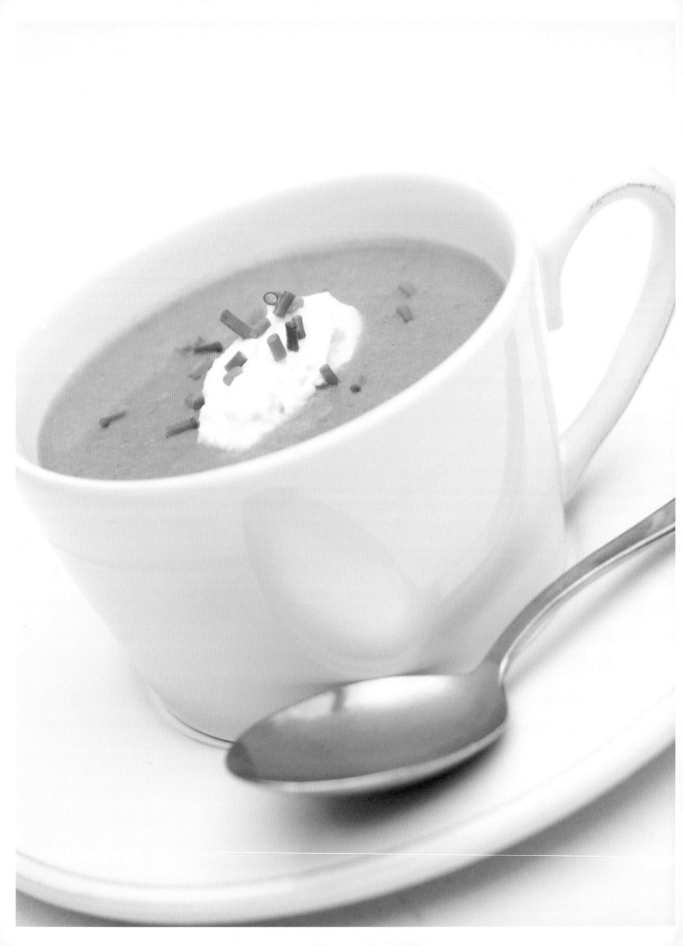

chestnut soup

serves 4

This is an elegant French classic and one of my favourites. Heaven in a cup. It's rich, creamy and light at the same time.

415g chestnut purée, 1 tin
1.2 litres chicken stock
salt & pepper
1¼ tsp sugar
zest of 1 lemon
large knob of butter
2 stalks celery, finely chopped
1 medium white onion, finely chopped
250ml milk, warmed
whipped cream for serving
a few chives, finely chopped

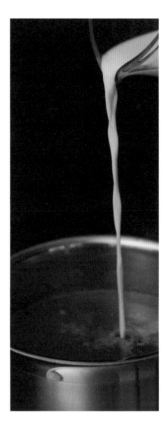

Cook the chestnut purée and stock in a deep pan on medium heat for about 20 minutes. Season to taste then add the sugar, lemon zest, butter, celery and onion. Allow to simmer for a further hour. The mixture should be soft enough to pass easily through a sieve. Adjust the thickness by adding half the warm milk before straining. Once strained, add sufficient milk to create a velvety texture. Serve warm with a dollop of whipped cream and sprinkle with chives.

Each portion provides 7g protein and 330kcals

nutrient	thumbs-up score
sodium	🔥🔥🔥🔥
chloride	🔥🔥
vitamin B6	🔥🔥
vitamin B12	🔥🔥
calcium	🔥🔥
copper	🔥
fibre (non-starch polysaccaride)	🔥
phosphorous	🔥
potassium	🔥

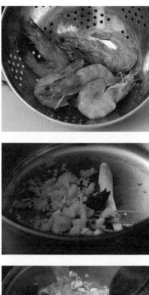

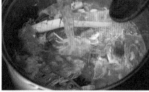

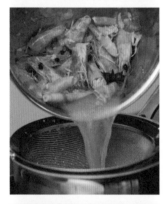

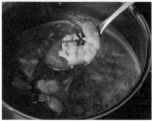

prawn & ginger soup
serves 4

This is a wonderfully quick and delicious soup. Ginger is known to help with nausea, while the prawns deliver flavour, texture and much needed trace elements.

12 whole prawns
1 clove garlic, finely chopped
2 stalks celery, finely chopped
5cm piece ginger, peeled
1 stalk lemon grass, bruised
1 star anise
fresh dill
500ml chicken stock
250ml water
1 bunch fresh chive
1 bunch fresh basil
salt & pepper
1 egg white (optional)

Chop half the ginger. Shell and de-vein the prawns. Put the shells and heads in a saucepan with the garlic, celery, chopped ginger, lemon grass, star anise and the stalks from the dill (save the sprigs). Pour in the stock and water, season lightly and simmer for 30 minutes.

Julienne the remaining ginger and finely chop the dill sprigs, chive and basil.

Next strain the liquid through a fine sieve into a clean pan. Add the prawns, ginger and herbs and simmer for a few minutes until the prawns are cooked. Season to taste.

Just before serving, gently beat the egg white with a fork but do not make it frothy. Pour into the hot soup and swirl with a fork to make threads. Serve immediately.

If you want a heartier soup add ramen noodles.

Each portion provides 6g protein and 33kcals

nutrient	thumbs-up score
vitamin B12	>👍👍👍👍
sodium	👍👍
chloride	👍👍

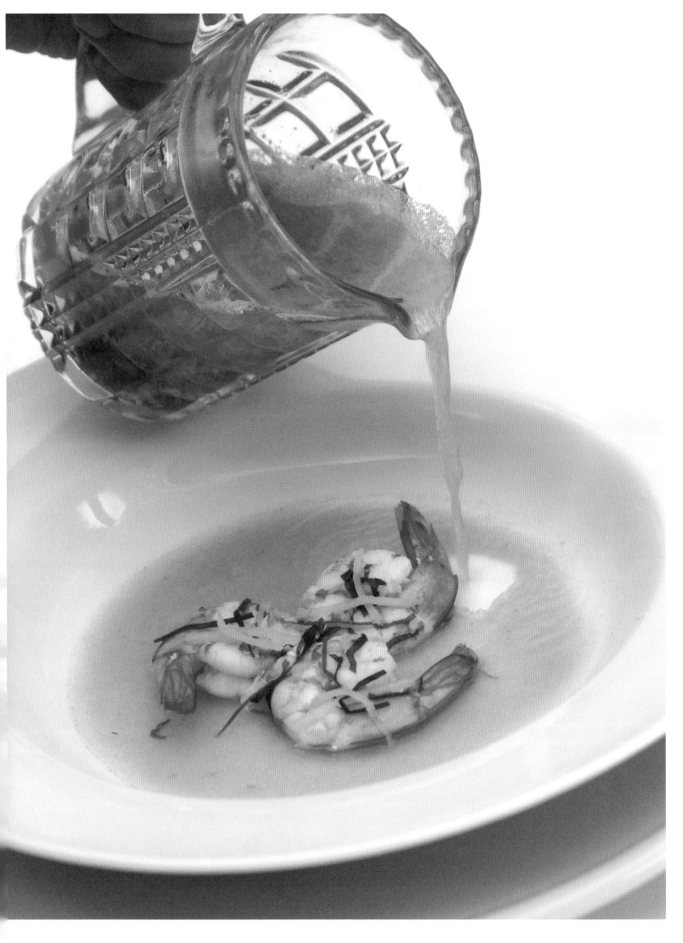

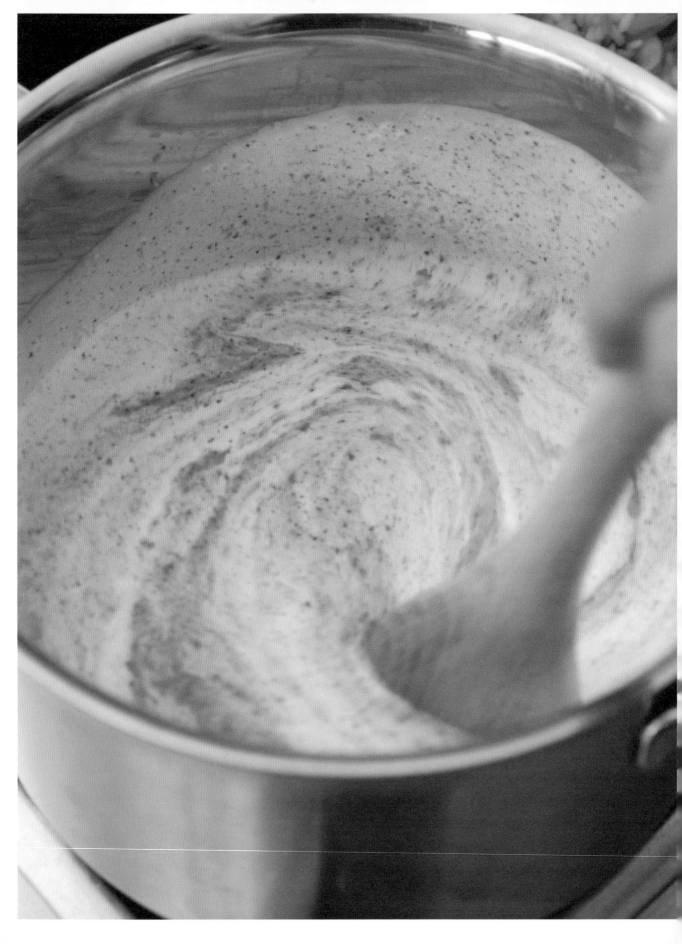

creamy watercress soup
serves 4

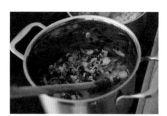

We are still learning about the power of watercress. If you want to enhance its natural peppery flavour, add a few drops of sriracha.

50g butter
450g leek, white only, washed and sliced
2 bunches watercress, chopped
1 medium potato, peeled and chopped
1 litre vegetable stock
150ml double cream
salt & pepper

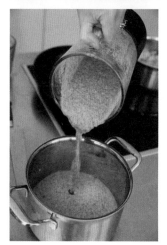

Melt the butter on a low heat in a deep, heavy saucepan. Add the vegetables (save a few watercress leaves for garnish) and sweat without colour until softened but still firm.

Pour in the stock and simmer on low heat for about 10 minutes. Remove from the heat and allow to cool. If the mixture is thicker than you want, add more stock. Liquidise the cooled soup. The mixture should be a dark, rich green. Set a small amount aside and return the rest to the saucepan.

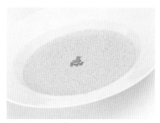

Now stir in the cream. Season to taste and reheat gently. To serve, ladle into a wide bowl then swirl some of the reserved dark soup around it.

Each portion provides 5g protein and 350kcals

nutrient	thumbs-up score
vitamin A (total retinol equivalents)	>👍👍👍👍
vitamin B6	>👍👍👍👍
vitamin C	>👍👍👍👍
sodium	👍👍
chloride	👍
thiamin	👍
calcium	👍
fibre (as non-starch polysaccharide)	👍
folate	👍
iron	👍
magnesium	👍
phosphorus	👍

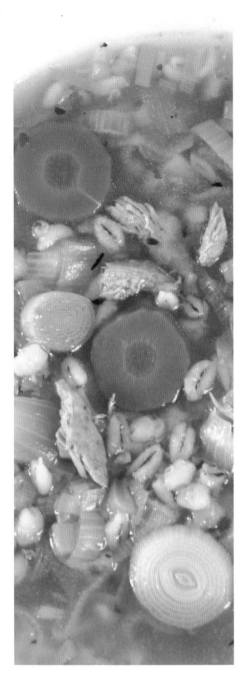

partridge cock-a-leekie soup

serves 4

There's something in the old wives tale about chicken soup being a great restorative. It's also a great source of iron so good when watching for anaemia.

6 partridge breasts

splash of olive oil

2-3 ltr chicken stock

1 leek, chopped

1 white onion, chopped

1 carrot, sliced

100g pearl barley

salt & pepper

marinade

50ml olive oil

100ml white wine

1 clove garlic, crushed

2 shallots, finely chopped

herbs de provençe

dash of sriracha

juice of 1 lemon

Allow breasts to marinate for 30 minutes then lightly brush them with olive oil and sear in a hot pan large enough to hold the soup. When cooked remove the breasts and allow them to rest. Take care, the breasts are small they cook quite quickly.

Return the pan to medium heat and deglaze the pan with a bit of chicken stock then add the chopped vegetables, barley and remainder of the stock and let simmer until the vegetables and barley are cooked but not too soft. Season to taste. Add more stock if required, as the barley will absorb a fair amount of moisture. Re-check the seasoning at this point.

Tear the partridge breasts into small pieces and add to the stock. Place on low heat and allow to simmer for another 30 minutes. Serve hot.

Each portion provides 38g and 471kcals

nutrient	thumbs-up score
iron	>👍👍👍👍
sodium	>👍👍👍👍
chloride	👍👍👍
phosphorus	👍👍👍
protein	👍👍👍
vitamin A (total retinol equivalents)	👍👍👍
vitamin B6	👍👍
magnesium	👍
potassium	👍
vitamin C	👍

potato & leek pottage
serves 4

This soup has soul. It is so nourishing and easy on digestion. The bright colour is tantalising and its creaminess makes it perfect comfort food.

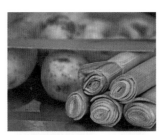

6-8 large floury potatoes
2-3 litres chicken or vegetable stock
dash of sriracha
1 egg yolk
3 leeks, whites only, finely chopped
1 tsp turmeric
½ tsp fennel seed
croutons*
fresh parsley, finely chopped
pinch of nutmeg
salt & pepper

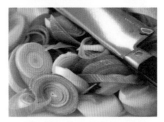

Peel and boil the potatoes in the stock with a drop of sriracha. Drain, reserving the stock, then purée with the egg yolk and nutmeg. Season to taste.

Sauté the leeks in olive oil until soft. Add half the potato purée, turmeric and fennel seed and whiz in a food processor gradually adding stock to achieve a creamy consistency. Season to taste and keep warm.

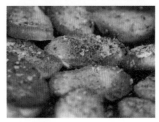

Pipe an island of potato purée into the centre of a bowl then surround with the leek pottage. Garnish with croutons, parsley and nutmeg. Serve hot.

Each portion provides 7g protein and 180kcals

*see *the basics*, page 280

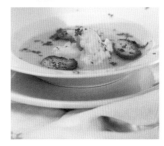

nutrient	thumbs-up score
vitamin B6	>👍👍👍👍
sodium	👍👍👍
chloride	👍👍👍
thiamin	👍👍
vitamin A	👍👍
vitamin C	👍
calcium	👍
iron	👍
phosphorus	👍
protein	👍

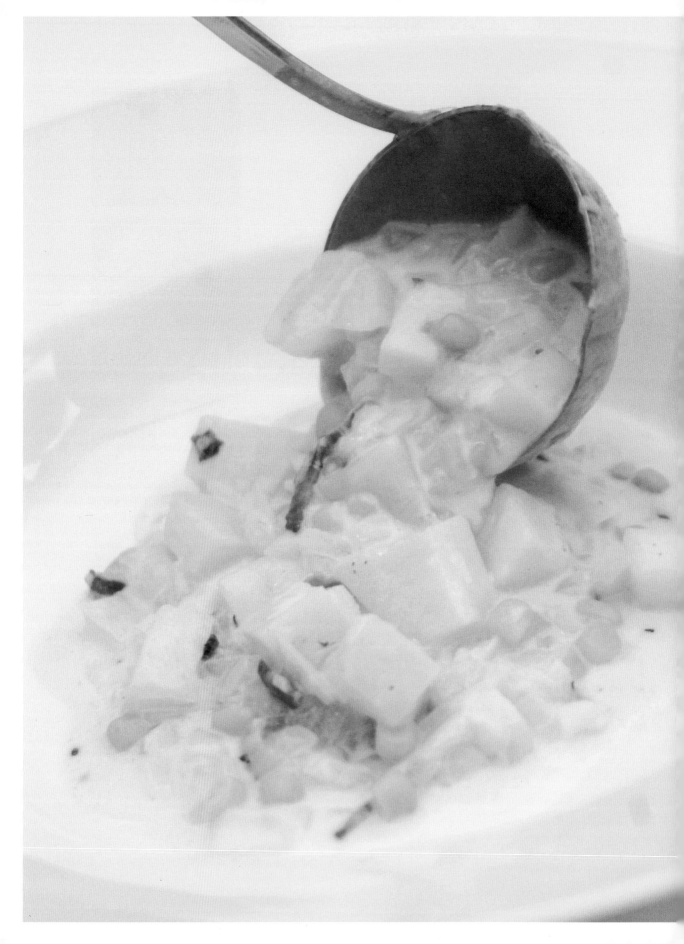

sage, sweetcorn & onion chowder
serves 4

This is a savoury gem. The sage, bacon and onion remain individual flavours that complement each other. A lovely warming dish.

60g butter

4 white onions, thinly sliced

200g sweetcorn

2 cloves garlic, crushed

4 smoked bacon rashers

2 tbsp flour

1 litre vegetable stock

300ml single cream

5 waxy potatoes, diced into fine cubes

1 tbsp fresh sage, finely chopped

2 tbsp white wine vinegar

sprigs of fresh sage

salt & pepper

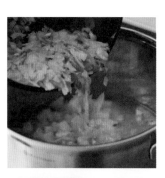

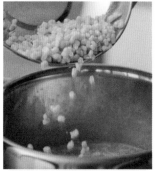

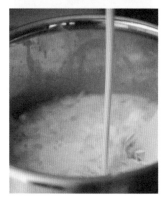

In a large frying pan, sauté the onions and garlic in butter ensuring to cook them without colour. Add the bacon and continue to sauté until cooked and the onions are slightly caramelised then stir in the flour and sauté for an additional minute and set aside.

Next place stock, onions and potatoes in a pot, season and simmer for about 20 minutes or until the potatoes are cooked but still firm. Add the cream and sweetcorn and bring back to the boil. Finally, add the sage and vinegar. Season to taste. Garnish with sage leaves and serve hot.

Each portion provides 14g protein and 530kcals

nutrient	thumbs-up score
sodium	>👍👍👍👍
chloride	👍👍👍👍
vitamin B6	👍👍👍👍
vitamin A total retinol equivalents)	👍👍
vitamin B12	👍👍
thiamin	👍👍
phosphorus	👍👍
calcium	👍
copper	👍
fibre (non-starch polysaccaride)	👍
folate	👍
potassium	👍
protein	👍

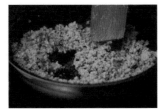

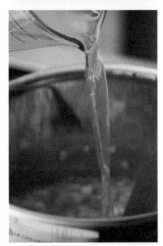

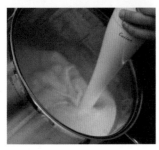

white bean, sausage & kale soup
serves 4

This soup is a bit of a 'big fella' and a real meal on its own. I'm always looking for ways to sneak a few more beans in.

350g extra-lean sausage meat

470g (2 tins) cannellini beans, drained and rinsed

1 tbsp olive oil

dash of sriracha

1 white onion, chopped

1 litre chicken stock

1 tbsp red wine vinegar

small bunch of curly kale or collards, finely chopped

salt & pepper

Brown the sausage meat in a lightly oiled pan.

Thoroughly rinse the beans, place them in a bowl and roughly mash.

Then in a lightly oiled deep, heavy pan, soften the onion and sriracha then add the stock and beans. Allow to simmer on medium heat for about 30 minutes then blitz with a hand blender until smooth. Pass the mixture through a sieve and return to the pot then stir in the vinegar and add the sausage. Bring to the boil to allow the soup to simmer for a further 30 minutes and season to taste. Finally add the chopped greens and cook on low heat until the greens are soft, about 30 minutes.

As the soup reduces and thickens add water to achieve desired consistency. Serve hot.

Each portion provides 24g protein and 320kcals

nutrient	thumbs-up score
vitamin A (total retinol equivalents)	>👍👍👍👍
vitamin C	>👍👍👍👍
sodium	>👍👍👍👍
chloride	>👍👍👍👍
fibre (non-starch polysaccaride)	👍👍👍
phosphorus	👍👍👍
vitamin B6	👍👍
folate	👍👍
calcium	👍👍
iron	👍👍
protein	👍👍
copper	👍
potassium	👍
magnesium	👍
zinc	👍

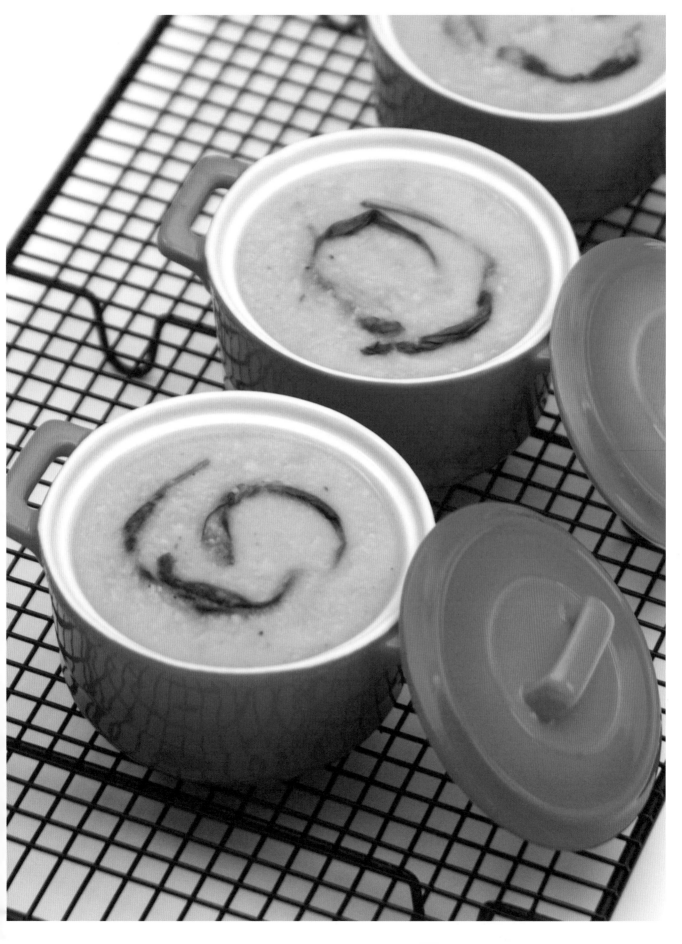

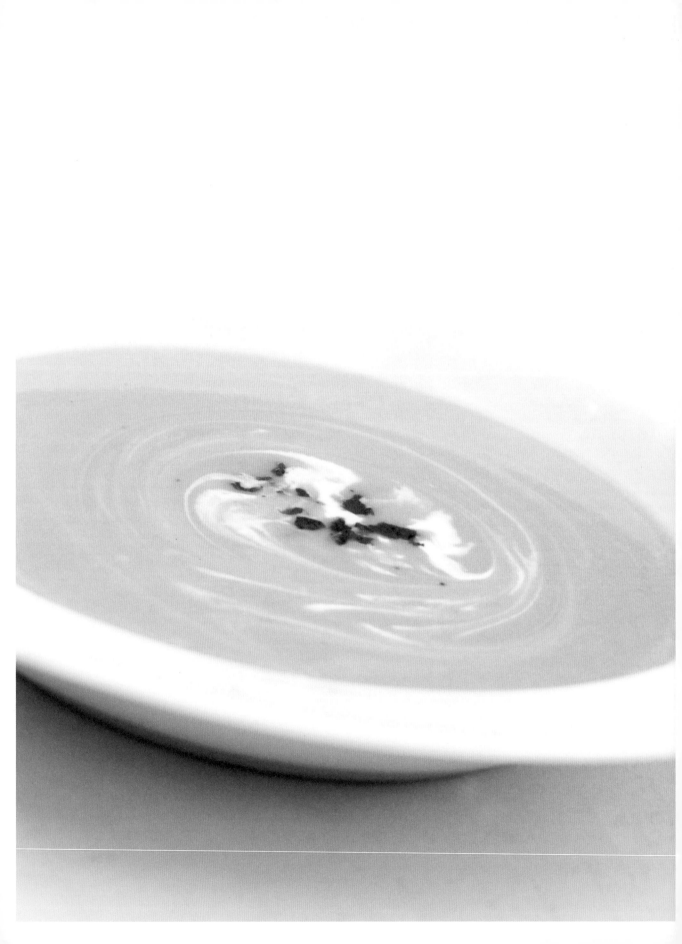

spicy pumpkin soup
serves 4

This is a lively soup that can wake up tired taste buds. The creaminess is easy on the tummy. It's also fast to prepare and freezes well.

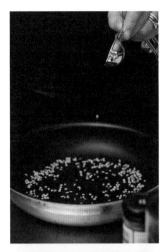

4 rashers smoked bacon

50g butter

dash of sriracha

1 medium onion, chopped

2 cloves garlic, chopped

900g pumpkin or butternut squash

1 tbsp coriander seeds

2 tsp cumin seeds

2 small dried chillies

1 litre chicken or vegetable stock

100ml coconut cream

salt & pepper

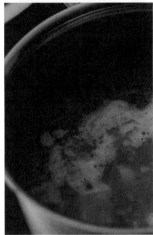

Fry the bacon until very crisp and break into bits. Set aside to use as garnish.

Melt the butter in a large saucepan, add the sriracha and cook the onion and garlic without colour.

Peel and seed the pumpkin. Remove the stringy bits as well. Chop into 2 inch cubes then add to the onion. Cook until the pumpkin is lightly golden and softening.

In a separate pan toast the coriander and cumin seeds over a low heat for about 2 minutes. They will release a lovely perfume. Place in a mortar, add the chillies and grind to a fine consistency. Add the spices to the pumpkin and cook for 1 minute.

Now add the stock and simmer for 20 minutes or until the pumpkin is tender.

Pour in most of the cream and blitz with a hand blender until smooth. Heat again until piping hot. Season to taste. Garnish with a drizzle of cream and bacon bits. Serve hot.

Each portion provides 11g and 280kcals

nutrient	thumbs-up score
vitamin B6	> 👍 👍 👍 👍
sodium	👍 👍 👍 👍
chloride	👍 👍 👍
thiamin	👍 👍
vitamin A	👍 👍
vitamin C	👍 👍
calcium	👍
iron	👍
phosphorus	👍
protein	👍

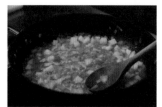

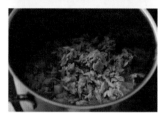

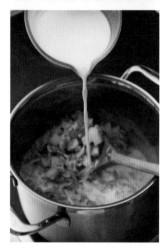

nova scotia clam chowder

serves 4

This maritime classic is a wonderfully warming meal and a great source of complete protein. The cream base makes it a good source of calcium. It's easy on the tummy too.

100g smoked bacon rashers

1 onion, chopped

1 stalk celery, chopped

350ml boiling water

4 medium waxy potatoes, diced

300g small clams, fresh or tinned (2 tins drained weight)

milk

120ml single cream

3 tsp butter

1 tsp celery salt

salt and pepper

Fry the bacon until crisp in a large saucepan then remove, dry and break into bits.

Next add the onions and celery to the drippings and cook without colour. Add the boiling water and potatoes and boil until just tender. This should take about 10 minutes. Drain the clams over a jug and top up the clam liquid with milk to make 1 litre and add this to the potatoes.

Gently heat to a simmer then add the clams, cooked bacon, cream, butter and seasoning. Heat until the broth is creamy. Be careful not to boil. Serve hot.

Each portion provides 22g protein and 300kcals

nutrient	thumbs-up score
vitamin B6	>👍👍👍👍
sodium	>👍👍👍👍
chloride	>👍👍👍👍
iron	👍👍👍
phosphorus	👍👍
vitamin B12	👍👍
copper	👍👍
protein	👍👍
vitamin A (total retinol equivalents)	👍
niacin	👍
thiamin	👍
calcium	👍
potassium	👍
zinc	👍

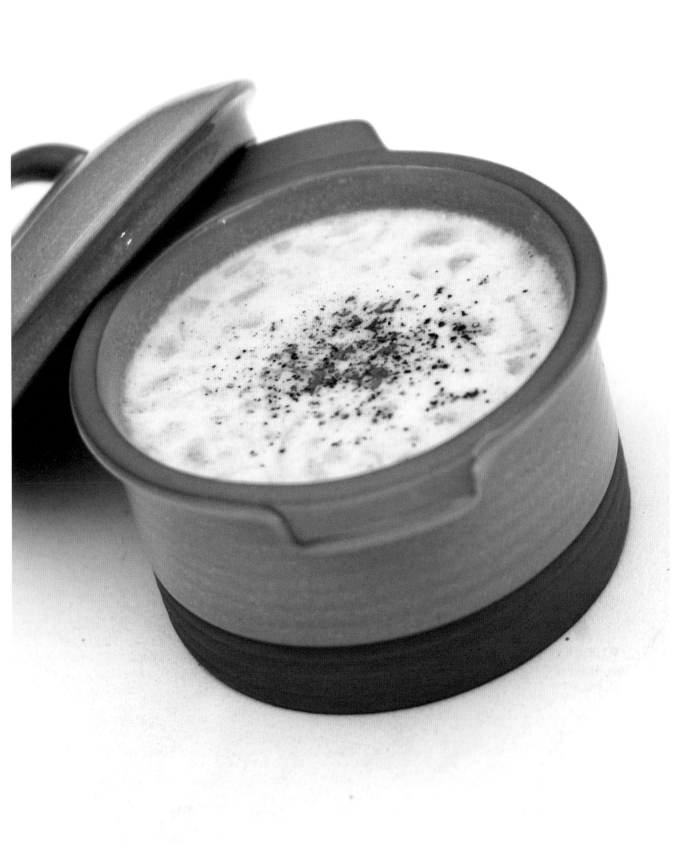

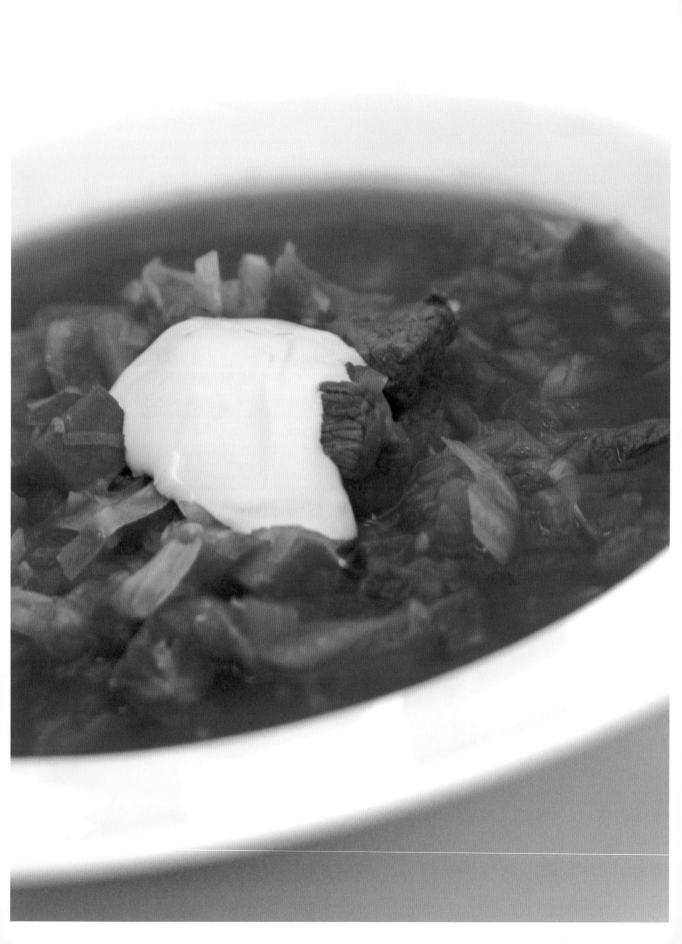

rich russian borscht

serves 4

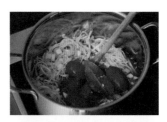

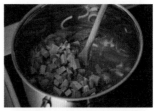

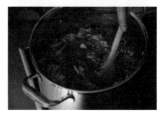

The beetroot gives this soup a sumptuous colour and it's packed with nutrition. It's a hearty dish.

½ small white cabbage
2 turnips
2 celery stalks, finely chopped
1 leek, white only, finely chopped
2 onions, finely chopped
500ml beef stock
1 tbsp red wine vinegar
1 tin whole italian tomatoes
1 bay leaf
salt & pepper
200g smoked ham
200g steak, diced
1 uncooked beetroot
200g sour cream
small bunch fresh dill, chopped

Shred cabbage and chop turnips, celery, leek and onions into small cubes. Place in a deep, heavy pan and add stock, vinegar, tomatoes and bay leaf. Bring to the boil and season to taste.

Next add the steak and lardons and simmer until the meat is tender. This will take about an hour.

Now peel and shred the raw beetroot and add to the soup. Allow to simmer for another 30 minutes. Check the seasoning again. Remove from heat and garnish with a dollop of sour cream and dill. Serve hot.

Each portion provides 27g protein and 300kcals

nutrient	thumbs-up score
vitamin B6	>👍👍👍👍
vitamin B12	>👍👍👍👍
sodium	>👍👍👍👍
chloride	👍👍👍👍
vitamin C	👍👍👍👍
phosphorus	👍👍👍
thiamin	👍👍
folate	👍👍
protein	👍👍
vitamin A (total retinol equivalents)	👍
niacin	👍
riboflavin	👍
calcium	👍
copper	👍
fibre (as non-starch	👍
iron	👍
magnesium	👍
potassium	👍
zinc	👍

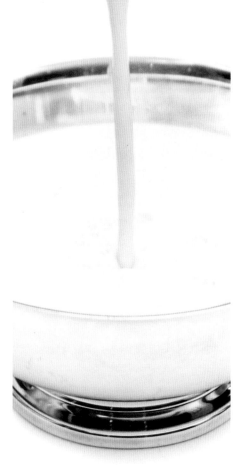

cream of cauliflower & cumin soup

serves 4

This soup is light and lovely anytime of year. It's a great and gentle way to get some essential vegetables and dairy.

3 onions, finely chopped
2 leeks, white only, finely sliced
550ml milk
salt & white pepper
nutmeg
1 clove garlic, crushed
1 tsp cumin seeds
1 head cauliflower, flowers only
100ml double cream
50g grated emmenthal

Warm garlic in oil in a large, heavy saucepan then add peeled and chopped onions and leeks and cook without colour. Add milk, salt and grate in some nutmeg. Put the cumin seeds in a small muslin sack* and suspend into the soup. Add the cauliflower and let simmer for 30 minutes.

Remove the cumin bag then liquidise the soup with a hand blender until smooth. If you want a very smooth, velvety soup pass it through a sieve then return to the heat to warm. Ladle hot soup into bowls, top with grated cheese and grill to melt the cheese.

Each portion contains 17g protein and 440kcals

* Paper egg-poaching sacks work well for this and can be bought at most supermarkets.

nutrient	thumbs-up score
vitamin B6	👍👍👍👍
vitamin B12	👍👍👍👍
vitamin C	👍👍👍👍
vitamin A (total retinol equivalents)	👍👍👍
calcium	👍👍👍
phosphorous	👍👍👍
folic acid	👍👍
thiamin	👍👍
iodine	👍👍
riboflavin	👍
copper	👍
fibre (as non-starch polysaccharide)	👍
iron	👍
magnesium	👍
potassium	👍
protein	👍
zinc	👍

cream of mushroom soup & herb crostini

serves 4

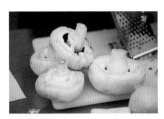

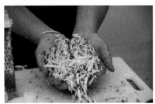

I simply love this soup. It can be made in a large batch and frozen in small portions.

800g chestnut and or cup mushrooms

1 medium red onion, finely chopped

2 shallots, finely chopped

1 clove garlic, smashed

olive oil

1 litre chicken or vegetable stock

250ml single cream

1 tbsp thyme leaves, finely chopped

dash of sriracha

salt & pepper

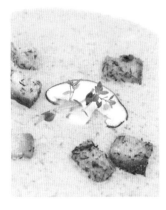

Grate the mushrooms with a cheese grater and finely chop the onions and shallots.

Next, lightly coat a large frying pan with olive oil then add the mushrooms. Leave on low heat and allow the mushrooms to fry until the moisture is gone. This will take 30-40 minutes. Add the onion, shallots, garlic and sriracha and thyme. Continue on low heat until the onions and shallots are cooked through.

Transfer the mushroom mixture into a deep, heavy pan with stock and bring to a simmer. Cover and let simmer for 20-30 minutes. Remove the cover and add cream. Continue to simmer until the soup is a nice consistency, not too watery but not too thick.

When ready blitz half of the mixture in a hand bender until smooth then return to the pot. Use vegetable stock or the jus from rehydrated dried mushrooms if you need to adjust thickness. Serve hot with herb crostini*.

Each portion provides 12g protein and 300kcals

*see *the basics*, page 284

nutrient	thumbs-up score
copper	>👍👍👍👍
sodium	👍👍👍👍
chloride	👍👍👍
vitamin B6	👍👍
riboflavin	👍👍
phosphorus	👍👍
selenium	👍👍
vitamin A total retinol equivalents)	👍
vitamin B12	👍
fibre (non-starch polysaccaride)	👍
folate	👍
niacin	👍
thiamin	👍
calcium	👍
iron	👍
potassium	👍
protein	👍

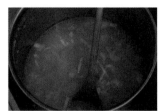

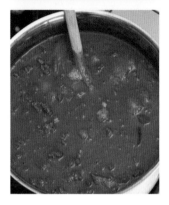

tuscan bean soup

serves 4

This soup is a grand Italian classic and with this many beans it has to be a best friend.

2 tbsp olive oil

dash of sriracha

2 cloves, garlic, peeled and crushed

2 onions, chopped

2 leeks, chopped

2 carrots, chopped

4 sprigs thyme

2-3 sprigs fresh rosemary

2 bay leaves

1 litre vegetable stock

juice of ½ lemon

400g chopped tomatoes, tinned are fine

1 tin cannellini beans, drained and rinsed

1 tin borlotti beans, drained and rinsed

4 links spicy italian sausage

bunch of parsley, chopped

salt & pepper

nutrient	thumbs-up score
vitamin A (total retinol equivalents)	>🔥🔥🔥🔥
vitamin B6	>🔥🔥🔥🔥
vitamin B12	🔥🔥🔥🔥
sodium	🔥🔥🔥🔥
chloride	🔥🔥🔥🔥
thiamin	🔥🔥🔥
iron	🔥🔥🔥
phosphorous	🔥🔥🔥
folate	🔥🔥
potassium	🔥🔥
protein	🔥🔥
zinc	🔥🔥
niacin	🔥
riboflavin	🔥
calcium	🔥
copper	🔥
magnesium	🔥
selenium	🔥

Heat oil in a deep, heavy saucepan and gently cook the garlic, onions, leeks and carrots until soft. Add thyme, rosemary and bay leaves, stock, lemon juice and tomatoes and simmer for 20 minutes. Add beans and some chopped parsley. Season to taste and continue to simmer for another 10 minutes.

In a separate pan grill sausages. When cooked, remove meat from casings, crumble then set aside.

Purée 1½ cups of the soup then re-introduce along with the sausage. Re-heat and check the seasoning. This will give the soup body without making it too thick.

Garnish with grated parmesan and serve with crusty bread.

Each portion provides 31g protein and 600kcals

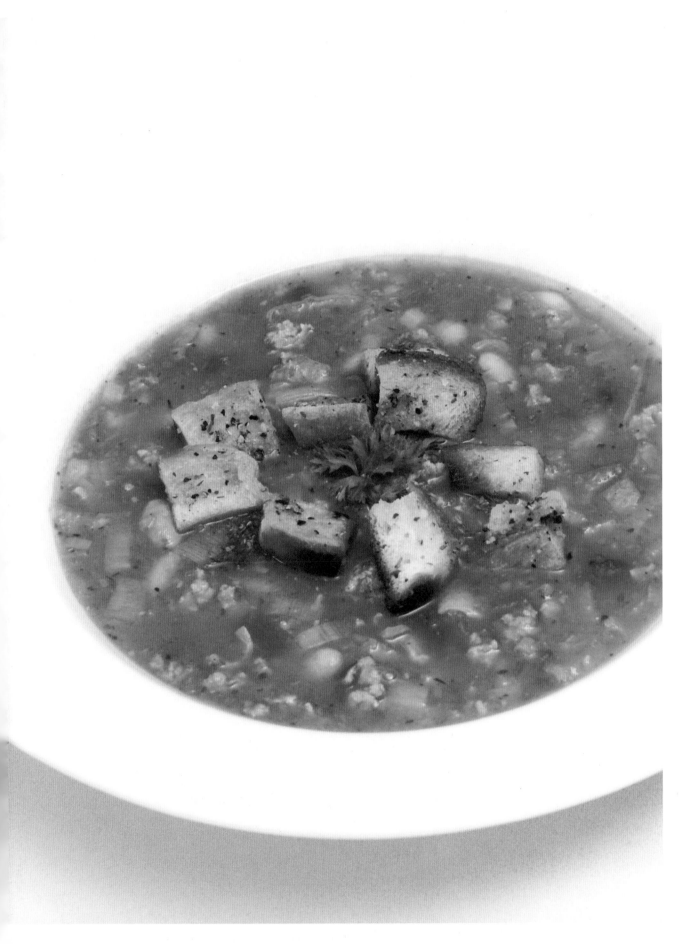

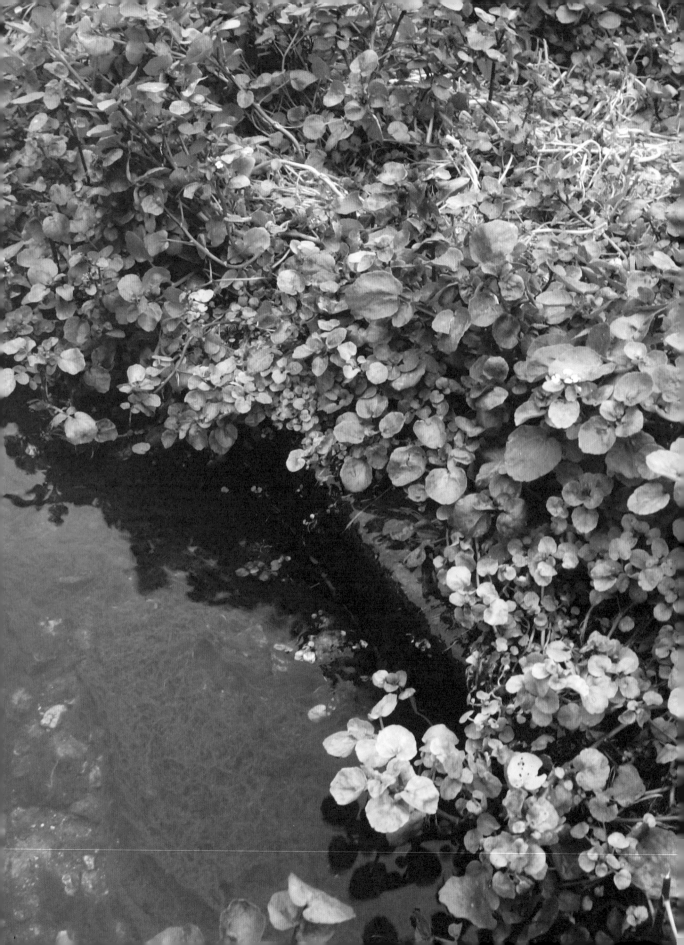

salads

salads

cesar	103
tabouleh	104
mediterranean fennel	105
greek salad	106
watercress & crispy shallot	109
beetroot & horseradish	110
ichiban slaw	111
potato	112
egg & tuna	114
cobb	115
spinach	117
roasted beetroot & goat's cheese	118

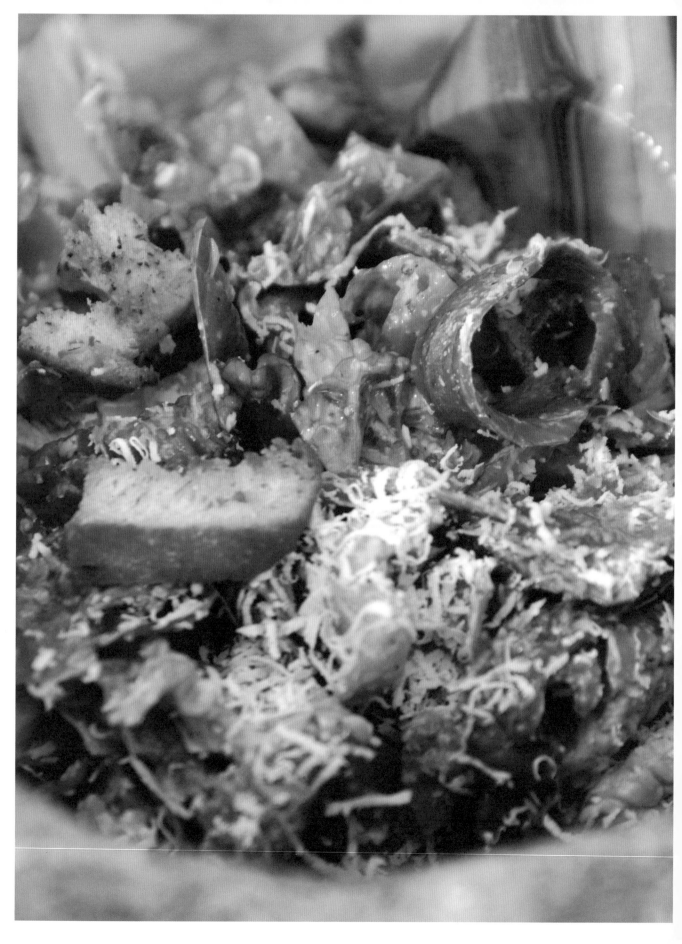

cesar salad

serves 4

This original recipe is a winner for vitamin B12 served on its own. It has wonderful crunchy texture and aroma and the strong flavours can really help wake up sleeping tastebuds.

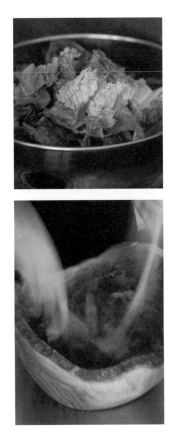

1 clove garlic, whole
2 heads romaine lettuce, torn
small anchovies
croutons*
½ cup parmesan cheese, finely grated
black pepper

dressing

2 cloves garlic, crushed
juice of 1 lemon
olive oil
2 egg yolks
1 tsp worcestershire sauce
1 tsp dry mustard
salt & pepper

Cut the garlic in two and rub the cut halves over the inside of a wooden salad bowl to season. Add the dressing ingredients and whisk together. Add the lettuce, anchovies and croutons and toss to combine. Sprinkle over the cheese and finish with a generous amount of black pepper.

Each portion provides 10g protein and 400kcals

*see the basics, page 280

nutrient	thumbs-up score:
vitamin B12	>👍👍👍👍
vitamin B6	👍👍
sodium	👍👍
chloride	👍👍
calcium	👍
phosphorus	👍

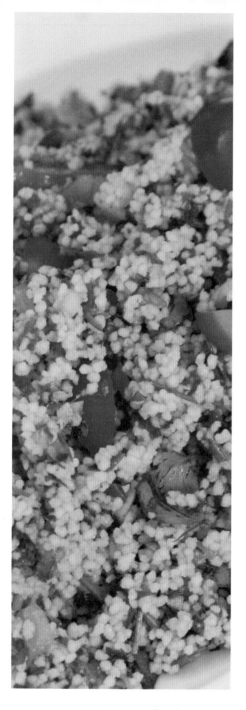

tabouleh

serves 6-8

Tabouleh is such a flexible salad and is an easy little snack as well as accompaniment to just about anything. The lemon gives it a freshness that can cut through those metal mouth days.

250g couscous
500ml chicken or vegetable stock
100ml olive oil
dash of sriracha
1 medium onion, finely chopped
3 italian tomatoes, chopped
1 bunch of flat leaf parsley, chopped
1 bunch of coriander, chopped
1 bunch of mint, chopped
2 tsp tomato purée
1 lemon, halved and seeds removed

Put the couscous in a bowl. Bring the stock to the boil then pour over the couscous and set aside.

Warm the oil in a frying pan, add the sriracha and onion and cook without colour. Add two of the chopped tomatoes, half the herbs and tomato purée. Season to taste and simmer gently without stirring. Do not let the mixture become too dry.

Fluff the couscous with a fork then stir in the remaining tomato, onion and herb mixture. Chop half the lemon (rind and all) and add to couscous with the remaining tomato and herbs. Sprinkle with the juice from the other half of the lemon and chill until ready to serve.

Each portion provides 6g protein and 390kcals

nutrient	thumbs-up score
vitamin B6	>👍👍👍👍
vitamin C	>👍👍👍👍
iron	👍👍
sodium	👍👍
vitamin A (total retinol equivalents)	👍
folate	👍
thiamin	👍
phosphorus	👍

mediterranean fennel salad

serves 4

Fresh, simple and crunchy. This is a great accompaniment for fish.

1 fennel bulb

6 breakfast radishes

handful of french beans

½ cucumber

a few fresh dill tops, finely chopped

zest of 1 lemon

1 tsp lemon juice

3 tbsp olive oil

salt & pepper

Finely shred the fennel, slice the radish and julienne the beans. Remove the seeds and slice the cucumber into small sticks. Mix the vegetables together adding the dill and lemon zest. Mix together the oil and lemon and a bit of seasoning and mix into the salad.

Each portion provides 1g protein and 15kcals

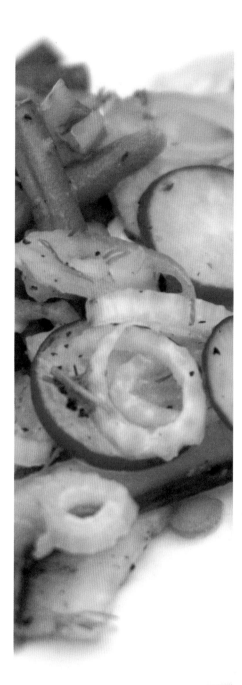

nutrient	thumbs-up score
sodium	👍
chloride	👍
vitamin C (18% RNI)	nearly 👍

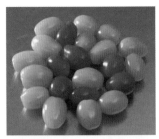

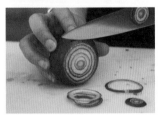

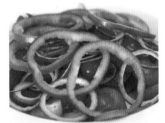

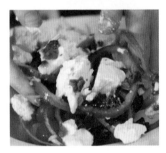

greek salad

serves 4

This is a salad to devour with your eyes. It is so bright and full of mouth-watering texture, aroma and flavour. To enhance this use a variety of tomatoes. It's full of vitamins and flavour.

600g tomatoes, baby plum, beef, vine-ripened italian

half a medium red onion, finely sliced

half a green pepper finely sliced

70g pitted black olives

juice of ½ lemon

200g of feta cheese

handful of fresh oregano

dressing

1 clove of garlic

2 tsp red wine vinegar

2 tsp olive oil

dash of sriracha

salt & pepper

Slice the tomatoes in various shapes. Choose a variety of tomatoes for colour and texture. Next add the onion and pepper rings squeeze olives into your hands and then drop into the salad crumble the feta cheese on top add lemon juice. Drizzle the dressing and top with the sprigs of oregano.

For the dressing, mash the garlic and add vinegar and oil. Season to taste.

Each portion provides 10g protein and 200kcals

nutrient	thumbs-up score:
vitamin B6	>👍👍👍👍
sodium	>👍👍👍👍
chloride	>👍👍👍👍
vitamin C	👍👍👍👍
vitamin A (total retinol equivalents)	👍👍
vitamin B12	👍👍
calcium	👍
folate	👍
phosphorus	👍

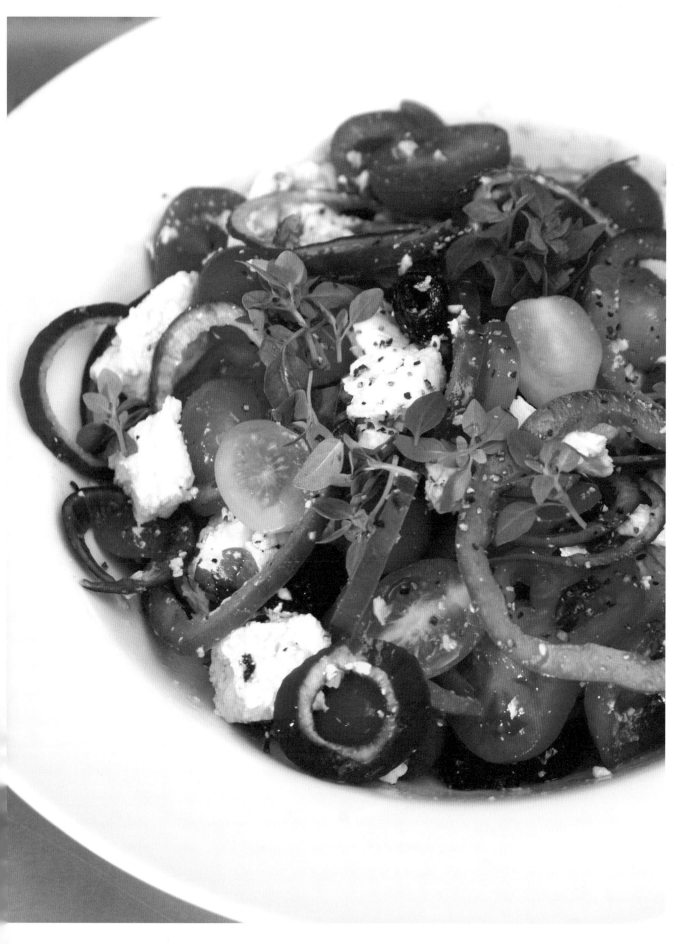

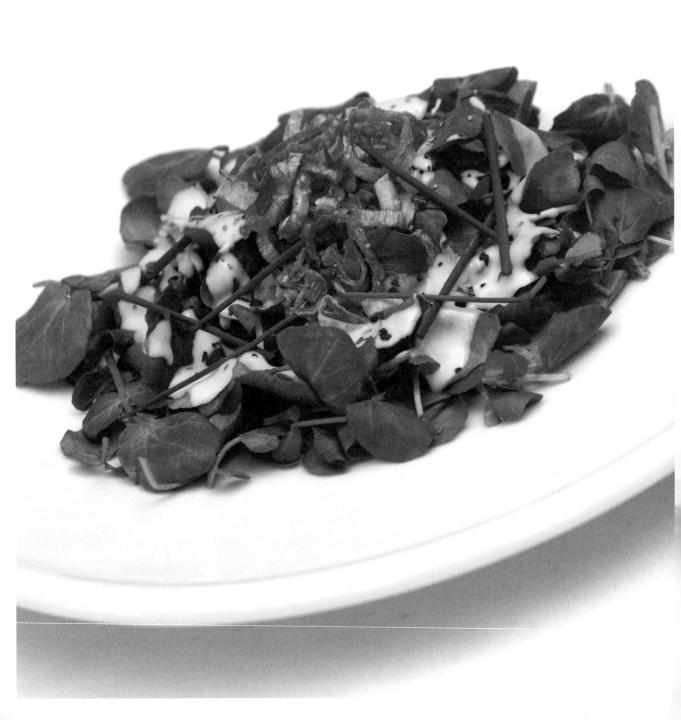

watercress & crispy shallot salad
serves 6-8

A super salad with big peppery and savoury flavour and is a great accompaniment for just about anything.

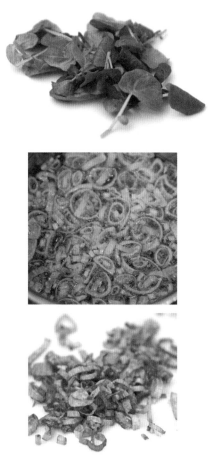

olive oil
5 large shallots, peeled and cut into rings
flour
milk
150g watercress, stalks removed

vinaigrette
3 tbsp olive oil
1 tbsp red wine vinegar
1 tbsp dijon mustard
1 tbsp créme fraiche
salt & pepper
a few chives, finely chopped

If you don't have a deep fat fryer, use a deep pan. Heat enough oil to deep-fry the shallot rings. Dip the rings in flour, then milk, then back in the flour and place in the oil with a slotted spoon. Fry until golden and crispy, then remove with the slotted spoon and place on paper towel to drain and cool.

In the meantime, prepare beds of watercress on plates, mix together the dressing ingredients and season to taste. Arrange the shallot rings on the salad, drizzle with dressing and garnish with spikes of chive.

Each portion provides 4g protein and 220kcals

nutrient	thumbs-up score
vitamin B6	>👍👍👍👍
vitamin C	👍👍
vitamin A (total retinol requirements)	👍
sodium	👍
chloride	👍

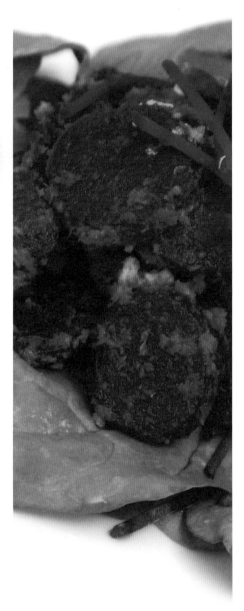

beetroot & horseradish salad

serves 4

The colour of this easy little number is simply wonderful. Adjust the amount of horseradish to suit your taste. It's bursting with flavour and packed with vitamin C.

400g small beetroot, cooked, peeled and sliced
75-100g beetroot leaves
juice of 1 lemon
2-3 tbsp hot horseradish
salt & pepper

If you are using raw beetroot, boil in heavily salted water until tender. Depending on the size of the beetroot this can take 1-2 hours. Make sure the water level is topped up to keep them submerged. Drain and rinse well (until water runs clear) and when cool, peel and slice. Leave one small beetroot behind to peel and julienne for added texture.

Place the beetroot slices in a mixing bowl and add lemon juice and horseradish. Toss gently and add a few julienne strips.

To serve, place the mixture on a bed of beetroot leaves and season to taste.

Each portion provides 3g protein and 50kcals

nutrient	thumbs-up score
vitamin C	👍👍
folate	👍👍
sodium	👍

ichiban slaw

serves 8

One of the great things about this cheeky little number is that it holds its body so it can be made in advance, chilled in a sealed container and served in small portions.

½ red or white cabbage, shredded
1 carrot, julienned
¼ cup almond slivers, lightly toasted
¼ cup sesame seeds, lightly toasted
1 pack dried ichiban noodles*

dressing

½ cup olive oil
2 tbsp white wine vinegar
1 tbsp sugar
salt & pepper
1 pack ichiban soup seasoning

In a large bowl, combine the cabbage, carrot, almonds and sesame seeds. Just before serving, break up the noodles and add to the cabbage mixture. Mix together the dressing ingredients, toss into the cabbage and set aside for one hour to allow the noodles to soften slightly. Serve chilled.

Each portion provides 3g protein and 230kcals

*any variety of ramen or packaged pot noodles works.

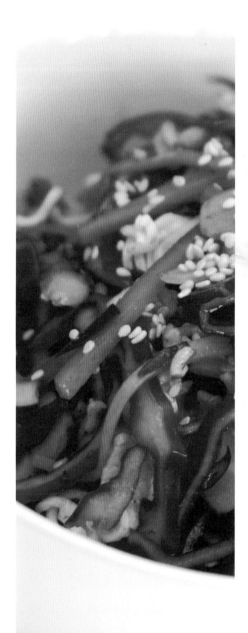

nutrient	thumbs-up score
vitamin A	19%
vitamin C	17%
phosphorous	16%
several nutrients come close reaching 20% RNI	

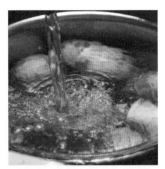

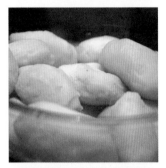

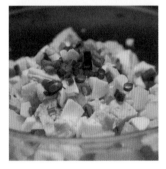

potato salad
serves 8

This salad can be made in advance and served in small portions. It's creamy and crunchy at the same time. The mustard and radishes give it a bit of extra kick.

10-12 medium potatoes, unpeeled
4 eggs, hard-boiled and chopped
2 stalks celery, finely diced
2 spring onions, finely diced
4 radishes, finely chopped
3 tbsp dried mustard
1 large jar mayonnaise
salt & pepper
1 tsp paprika

Boil the potatoes whole until they are cooked but not soft. Run under cold water to halt the cooking process, then peel. Cut into large cubes.

Add the rest of the ingredients and mix. Season to taste. Go carefully with the mayonnaise, most recipes call for too much. Refrigerate. Serve chilled.

Each portion provides 13g protein and 1100kcals

nutrient	thumbs-up score
vitamin B6	>👍👍👍👍
vitamin B12	>👍👍👍👍
sodium	👍👍👍
chloride	👍👍👍
vitamin A total retinol equivalents)	👍👍
iodine	👍👍
phosphorus	👍👍
vitamin C	👍
folate	👍
riboflavin	👍
thiamin	👍
copper	👍
iron	👍
potassium	👍
protein	👍
zinc	👍

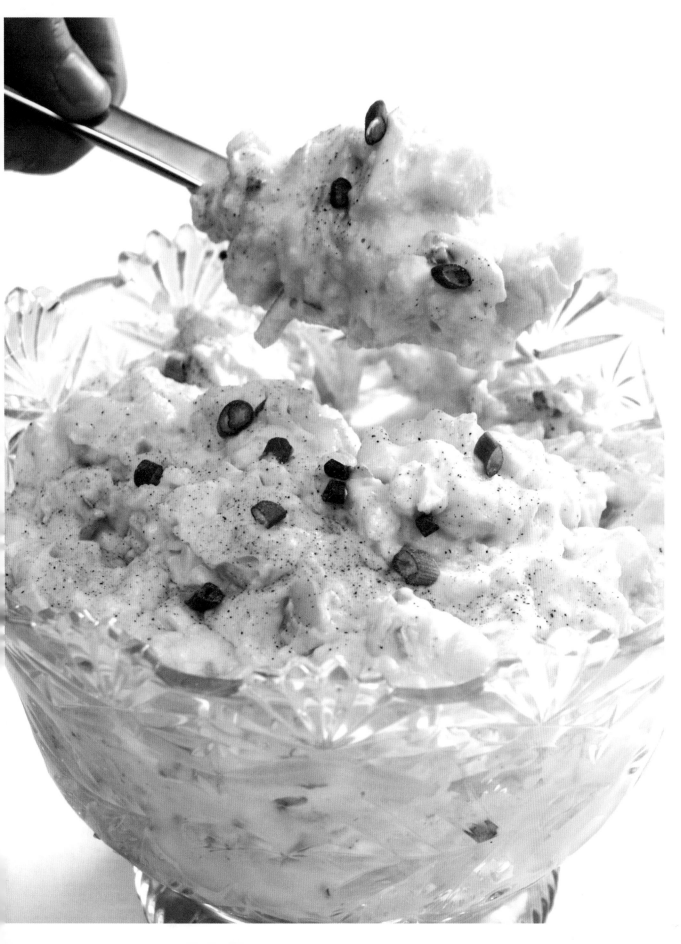

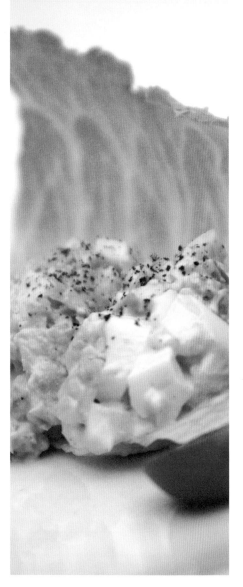

nutrient	thumbs-up score:
vitamin B6	>👍👍👍👍
vitamin B12	>👍👍👍👍
iodine	👍👍
selenium	👍👍
sodium	👍👍
chloride	👍👍
vitamin A (total retinol equivalents)	👍
folate	👍
niacin	👍
riboflavin	👍
fibre (non-starch polysaccaride)	👍
iron	👍
phosphorus	👍
protein	👍

egg & tuna salad
serves 4

An old-fashioned egg and tuna salad is the ultimate Saturday sandwich. Add sweetcorn if you must. So often these simple recipes win the day.

egg salad

4 free range, organic eggs

¼ cup mayonnaise

1 tsp mustard powder

½ stick celery, finely chopped

paprika

salt & pepper

Hard boil the eggs then run under cold water for 1 minute before peeling. Dice into course chunks and add celery, mustard and mayonnaise and a pinch of paprika. Mix together, season to taste and garnish with a further sprinkle of paprika.

tuna salad

130g tuna, 1 tin drained weight

1 egg, hard-boiled

1 spring onion, finely chopped

½ stick celery, finely chopped

¼ cup mayonnaise

salt & pepper

iceberg lettuce for serving

toast

Thoroughly rinse the tuna from can until water runs clear. Then pat dry. Chop the egg into small but not tiny bits. Add all ingredients in a bowl and season to taste.

Serve a scoop of both salads with lettuce as a small bite or on toast as a sandwich.

Each portion provides 13g protein and 250kcals

cobb salad

serves 4

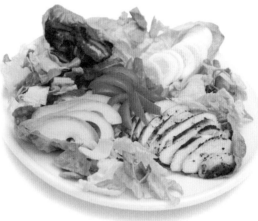

The all-American salad! Loads of flavours in small portions and nearly every bit of nutrition and dietary help money can buy. The dressing is sensational!

smoked bacon rashers

1 chicken fillet

½ head romaine lettuce

½ head iceberg lettuce

1 small bunch curly endive

½ bunch of watercress, stems removed

2 ripe avocados

1 tomato, seeds removed and finely chopped

2 eggs, hard boiled, yolk and white separated and finely chopped

2 tbsp fresh chives, chopped

roquefort dressing

⅓ cup red wine vinegar

1 tbsp dijon mustard

⅔ cup olive oil

½ cup roquefort, finely crumbled

1 tsp sugar

salt & pepper

Fry the bacon until crisp and drain on a paper towel. When cool, crumble to make crispy bits. Season the chicken and grill until cooked through. Allow to rest for 10 minutes then slice.

Peel and dice the avocados. In a large bowl, toss together the lettuce and watercress. Lay onto plates then top with chicken, bacon, tomato, avocado and eggs and sprinkle with chives.

For the dressing, whisk together the vinegar and mustard and season to taste. Add the oil in a slow stream and whisk until emulsified. Stir in the roquefort. Add the sugar to taste. Be careful not to over-sweeten. Serve the dressing on the side.

Each portion provides 34g protein and 940kcals

nutrient	thumbs-up score
vitamin B6	>👍👍👍👍
sodium	>👍👍👍👍
chloride	👍👍👍👍
vitamin B12	👍👍👍
thiamin	👍👍👍
phosphorus	👍👍👍
protein	👍👍👍
niacin	👍👍
vitamin A (total retinol equivalents)	👍
vitamin C	👍
riboflavin	👍
calcium	👍
copper	👍
fibre (as non-starch polysaccharide)	👍
folate	👍
iron	👍
magnesium	👍
potassium	👍
selenium	👍
zinc	👍

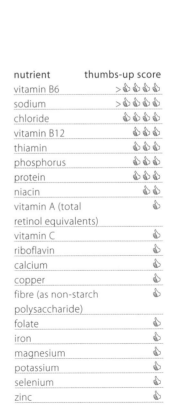

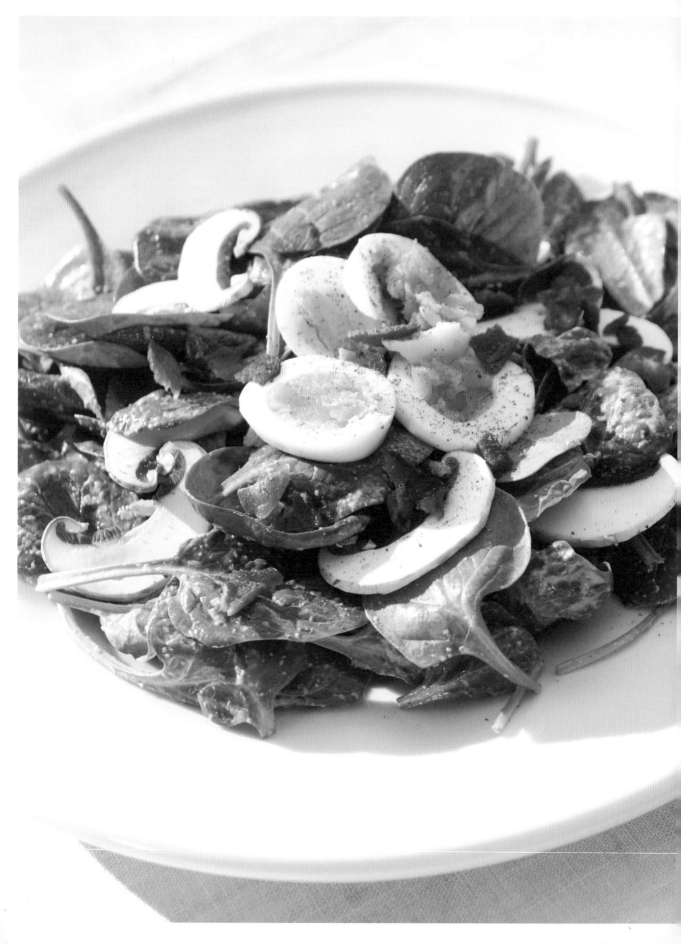

spinach salad
serves 4

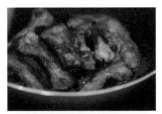

This recipe is based on the original classic. The bacon bits pop up like little nuggets of happiness. Uncooked spinach provides a healthy daily portion of iron so it's good when watching for anemia.

young spinach leaves
2 eggs, hard-boiled and sliced
4 rashers crisp streaky bacon, grilled and crumbled
4 button mushrooms, finely sliced

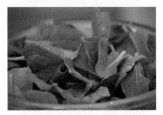

dressing

1 tbsp grainy dijon mustard
1 handful fresh basil, chopped
1 tsp coarsely cracked black pepper
2 large shallots, finely chopped
2 egg yolks
80ml balsamic vinegar
250ml olive oil
dash of worcestershire sauce
salt & pepper

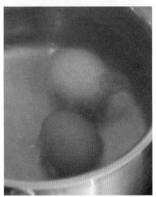

Place the mustard, basil, black pepper, shallots, egg yolks, worcestershire sauce and vinegar in a blender. Blend on a high speed and slowly add the oil. Add a little water if the mixture becomes too thick. Season to taste with the remaining ingredients. One helpful hint is that if the vinegar overpowers the dressing you can add a little sugar to balance the flavour.

Wash and dry the spinach leaves and lay out on a plate. Add the sliced egg, bacon and mushrooms and drizzle with dressing.

Each portion provides 12g protein and 620kcals

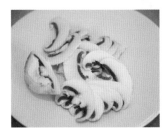

nutrient	thumbs-up score
vitamin B6	>👍👍👍👍
vitamin A (total retinol equivalents)	👍👍👍
vitamin B12	👍👍👍
sodium	👍👍👍
chloride	👍👍👍
folate	👍
iodine	👍
iron	👍
phosphorus	👍
protien	👍

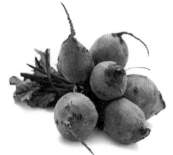

roasted beetroot & goat's cheese salad

serves 6

I think this is a real beauty. The colour is lovely. The flavour mixture is divine and it's so very easy to prepare.

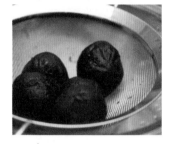

8 baby beetroot, rinsed and trimmed

1 tbsp olive oil

salt & pepper

1 shallot, julienned

dijon vinaigrette*

10 cups mesclun salad†

250g goat's cheese, cubed

handful of walnuts or pecans

Preheat oven to 200°Cf.

Place the beetroot in a roasting tin, drizzle with the olive oil and season. Cover with foil and roast for 25 minutes, then uncover and roast for a further 15 minutes or until fork-tender. Allow the beetroots to cool then peel, slice and place in a medium bowl with the shallot and drizzle with dijon vinaigrette.

Place on a bed of mesclun salad and top with goat's cheese. Sprinkle with walnuts or pecans and serve.

If you don't want to pfaff about with the beetroot, buy pre-cooked and rinse well.

Each portion provides 18g protein and 545kcals

*see *the basics*, page 282
†see *the basics*, page 281

nutrient	thumbs-up score
vitamin B6	👍👍👍👍
sodium	👍👍👍
chloride	👍👍👍
vitamin C	👍👍
folate	👍👍
phosphorus	👍👍
vitamin A total retinol equivalents)	👍
vitamin B12	👍
riboflavin	👍
calcium	👍
copper	👍
iodine	👍
magnesium	👍
protein	👍
iron	👍
zinc	👍

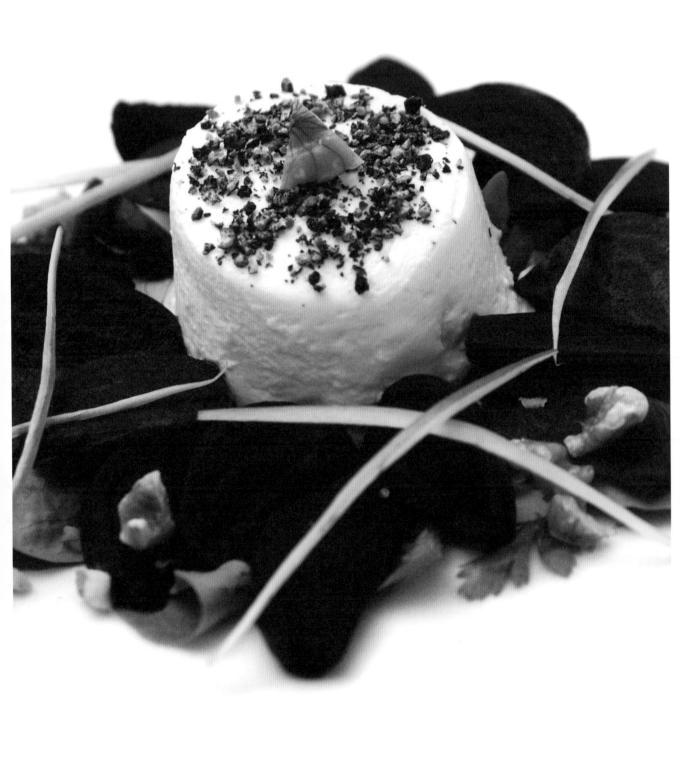

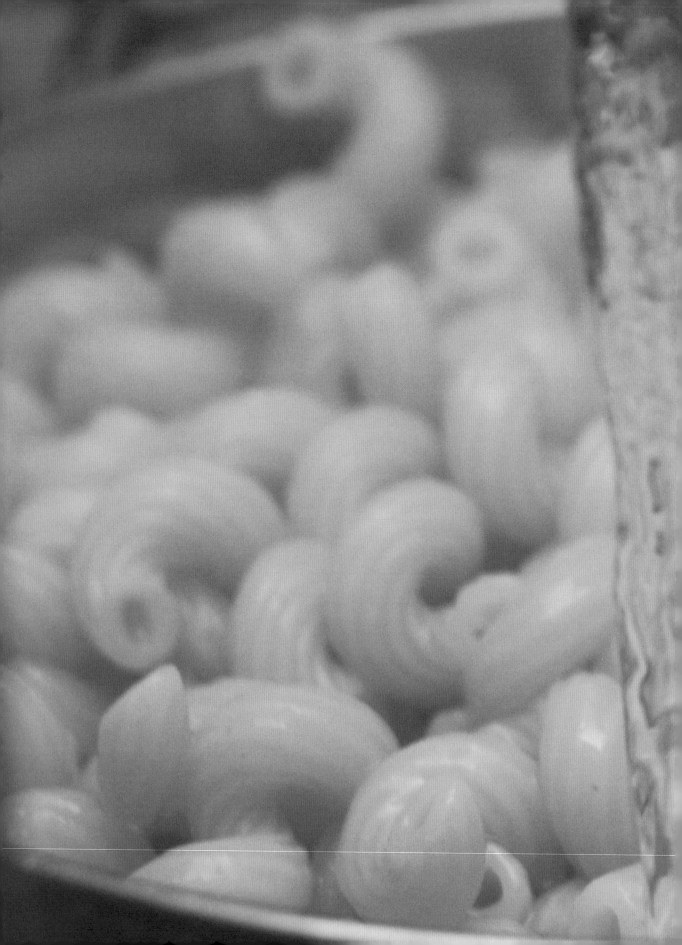

pizza, pasta
& risotto

pizza, pasta & risotto

pizza basics	124
pizza dough	124
tomato sauce & toppings	126
caramelised onion & truffle pizza	127
smoked alaskan salmon & caviar fettuccini pasta	129
penne pesto	130
old-fashioned tuna casserole	131
crab claw linguini with french beans & broad bean pesto	132
spaghetti carbonara	134
wild mushroom pappardelle in truffle cream	135
dijon & four cheese macaroni	137
angel hair ragu	138
creamy beetroot risotto	141
smoked haddock with pea & baby leek	142

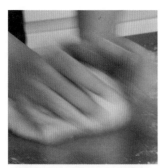

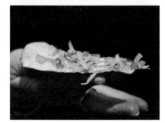

pizza basics
serves 4

I use pizza stones that allow the crust to be thin and crispy.

pizza dough
15g fresh yeast with a splash of warm water, (1½ tsp dried)

250g flour, type 00 hard durum wheat or strong bread

1 tsp salt

50ml olive oil

Preheat oven to 220°Cf. The pizza stones need to be heated for 45 minutes to an hour in advance.

Sift the flour and salt into a large mixing bowl and make a well in the middle. Drizzle in the oil and add the yeast. Mix with a wooden spoon, adding splashes of water as required, to make a soft dough. Turn out onto a floured surface and knead for 10-12 minutes until smooth and elastic. Split the dough into 2 balls and place in a lightly oiled bowl, giving each ball a light coating of oil. Cover and leave in a warm place for about 1½ hours.

Flatten out the dough and knead again on a lightly floured surface for 2-3 minutes. At this stage you can wrap the dough and freeze for future use.

Roll out the dough very thin. Take the pizza stone out of the oven, lightly flour the surface then lay the dough on the stone. Roll up the edge and sprinkle with salt. Allow the crust to bake on the stone for 1 minute then brush with a fine film of olive oil. You are now ready to add pizza sauce and toppings.

nutrient	thumbs-up score
vitamin B6	>👍👍👍👍
sodium	👍👍👍
chloride	👍👍👍
vitamin C	👍
riboflavin	👍
calcium	👍
copper	👍
fibre (as non-starch polysaccharide)	👍
folate	👍
iron	👍
phosphorus	👍
protein	👍

Our analysis has been done on basic pizza without the extra toppings so the extras are a nutritional bonus!

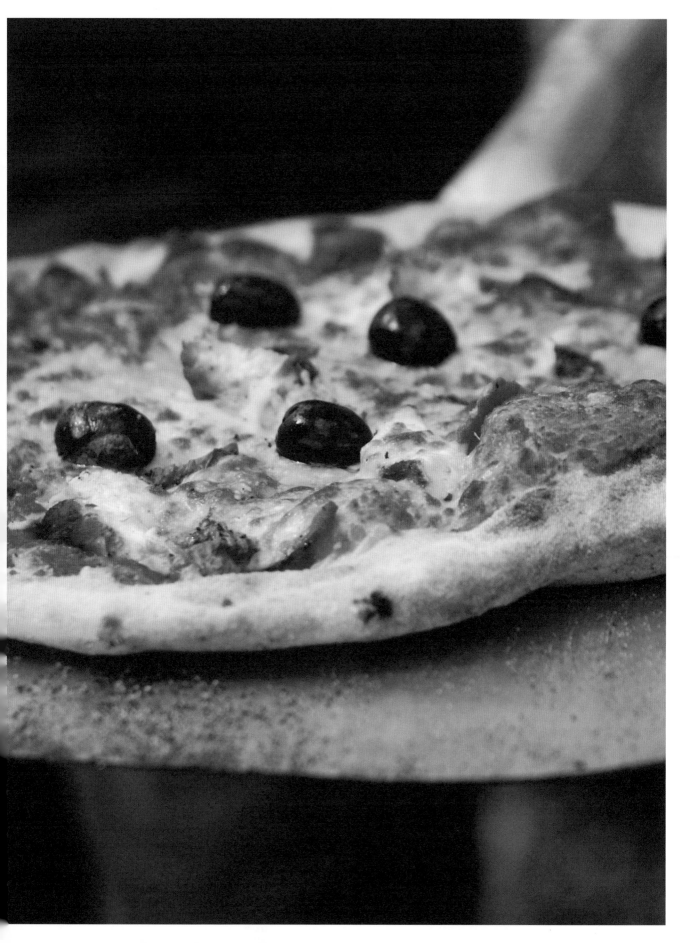

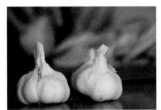

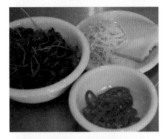

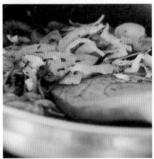

pizza sauce

2 tsp olive oil

2 large cloves garlic, crushed

dash of sriracha or 1 jalapeno pepper, finely chopped

1 medium onion, finely chopped

1 tin tomatoes or 4-6 italian tomatoes, chopped

1 tbsp tomato purée

herbs de provençe

250ml red wine

salt & pepper

Warm the garlic and the sriracha or pepper in a pan lightly coated with olive oil. Add the onion and cook until transparent. Add the tomatoes, purée, herbs, salt and pepper and a generous amount of red wine. Leave to simmer and reduce for at least an hour, stirring regularly. As the sauce thickens, add more wine. Once the sauce has achieved a nice rich consistency, set aside to cool.

toppings

a few favourites:

• sauteed artichoke hearts and mushrooms in garlic and wine

• caramelised onions, slice into thin rings and fry in oil until brown

• roasted peppers, skins removed, with dollops of goat's cheese

• pineapple and ham.

Avoid raw vegetables such as bell peppers, onions, mushrooms and fatty meats as the additional moisture can make the crust soggy.

Each portion provides 10g protein and 415kcals

caramelised onion & truffle

serves 4

This is a super pizza with bags of flavour if tomatoes are too acidy. It's a morish nibble and fab hors d'ouvres.

1 onion, unskinned

4 sprigs rosemary

4 sprigs thyme

2 bay leaves

3 garlic cloves, unpeeled

1 italian white truffle or truffle purée

225g mozzarella cheese, torn into pieces

225g gruyere cheese, grated

225g parmesan cheese, grated

small wild rocket leaves

In an oiled baking tray, slowly roast the onion with the rosemary, thyme, bay leaves and garlic cloves until onions are golden on the outside and soft to the touch. Peel the onion and garlic and mix into a rough purée.

Brush a thin film of oil over the pizza base. Spread the onion purée on the dough then grate over the truffle or dot with truffle purée. Sprinkle over the cheeses and bake. Top with a few leaves of rocket and serve hot.

Each portion provides 48g protein and 645kcals

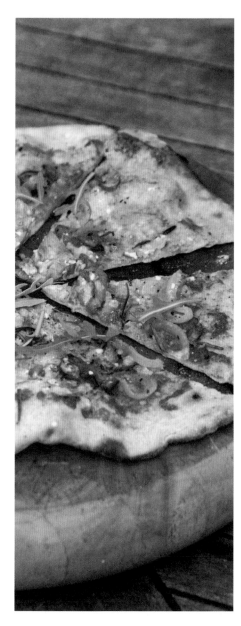

nutrient	thumbs-up score
vitamin B12	>👍👍👍👍
calcium	>👍👍👍👍
phosphorus	>👍👍👍👍
vitamin A(total retinol equivalents)	👍👍👍👍
protein	👍👍👍👍
sodium	👍👍👍👍
chloride	👍👍👍👍
zinc	👍👍👍
riboflavin	👍👍
copper	👍👍
vitamin B6	👍
folate	👍
iodine	👍
magnesium	👍

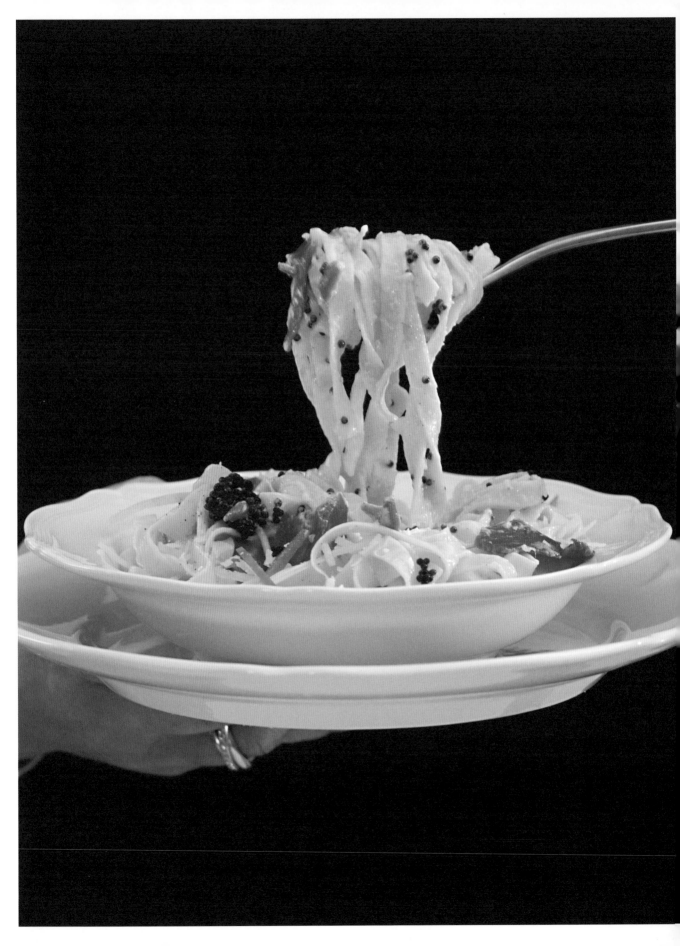

smoked alaskan salmon & caviar fettucini

serves 4

This is elegant and simple pasta that smiles. It always seems to say, 'I'm special.' The textures are simply wonderful.

1 knob butter
1 clove garlic, finely sliced
1 shallot, finely chopped
85ml white wine
175ml whipping cream
225g fettuccine
1 carrot, ½ leek & 1 stick celery, julienned
100g smoked alaskan salmon
100g parmesan cheese, grated
1 pinch nutmeg
1 pinch cayenne pepper
salt & pepper
jar of lumpfish caviar

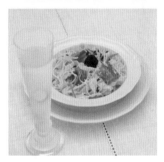

Boil the pasta in salted water to al dente.* Drain, rinse thoroughly and set aside.

Next sauté the garlic and shallots in butter. Cook without colour for 2 minutes then add the white wine and reduce by two-thirds. Add the cream and boil for 2 minutes. When ready to serve add the fettuccine, julienne of vegetables and salmon to the sauce, combine and turn the heat down low.

Just before serving, turn the heat back up, bring to a boil, season to taste and add half the parmesan cheese, the nutmeg and cayenne pepper. Garnish with a dollop of caviar and the rest of the parmesan.

Each portion provides 25g protein and 495kcals

*see *the basics*, page 280

nutrient	thumbs-up score
vitamin A (total retinol equivalents)	>👍👍👍👍
vitamin B12	>👍👍👍👍
sodium	👍👍👍👍
chloride	👍👍👍👍
vitamin B6	👍👍👍
phosphorus	👍👍👍
calcium	👍👍
copper	👍👍
protein	👍👍
riboflavin	👍
iodine	👍
selenium	👍
zinc	👍

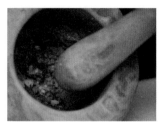

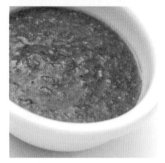

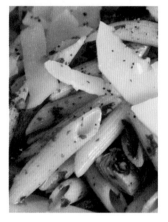

penne pesto

serves 4-6

Served warm or cold this is a super dish to prepare in advance. It also travels well so can be a nutritious meal on treatment days.

25g pine nuts, toasted

1 tsp salt

3 garlic cloves

leaves from 2 large bunches basil

150ml extra virgin olive oil

50g parmesan cheese, grated

dash of sriracha

freshly cracked black pepper to taste

500g penne

150g olive oil

1 garlic clove

dash of sriracha

1 tin small artichoke hearts, sliced

200g mushrooms, sliced

250ml white wine

herbs de provençe

30g black olives, stoned and halved

6 sun dried tomatoes in oil, chopped

150g parmesan cheese, shaved

nutrient	thumbs-up score
vitamin B12	>👍👍👍👍
copper	>👍👍👍👍
phosphorus	>👍👍👍👍
calcium	👍👍👍👍
iodine	👍👍👍👍
protein	👍👍👍
sodium	👍👍👍
chloride	👍👍👍
vitamin A total retinol equivalents)	👍👍
iron	👍👍
selenium	👍👍
zinc	👍👍
vitamin B6	👍
riboflavin	👍
magnesium	👍
potassium	👍

For the pesto pound the pine nuts, salt, garlic and a few basil leaves together in a mortar to create a silky paste. Put the paste and the rest of the ingredients in a food processor and blend until smooth. The paste should be rich green and quite dense in texture.

Cook the penne to al dente* then rinse and place in a large bowl.

Warm the garlic and sriracha in a lightly oiled pan then saute the artichokes and mushrooms with the wine, herbs and seasoning. Pour the mixture over the pasta, add the olives and tomatoes and toss to combine before stirring in the pesto. Season to taste and garnish with parmesan shavings.

Each portion provides 37g protein and 1380kcals

*see *the basics*, page 280

old-fashioned tuna casserole

serves 4

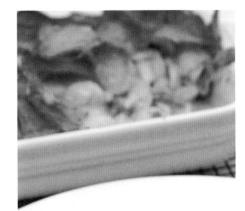

This all-American classic is famous for its ease and economy. It's a nutritious powerhouse and a fast way to feed the family. It's also famous for being a dish that you would bring to an ailing friend.

400g dry pasta (orecchiette is great)

370g flaked tuna, 2 tins, drained, rinsed and dried

500ml condensed cream of mushroom soup, 2 tins

knob of butter

1 medium onion, finely chopped

6 medium cup mushrooms, sliced

½ green pepper, finely chopped (optional)

200g petit pois

350g cheddar, grated

225g lightly salted crisps

Preheat oven to 180°Cf.

Boil the noodles in salted water until fully cooked then drain, rinse and set aside.

Next sauté the onion, mushrooms and pepper in butter until soft.

In a large bowl add the soup, tuna, sautéed vegetables, peas and noodles and mix. Place these in a deep casserole and cover with cheese and top with crisps. Bake for about 20 minutes, until hot and golden on top and serve.

Each portion provides 67g protein and 1360kcals

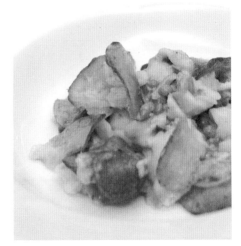

nutrient	thumbs-up score
vitamin B6	>👍👍👍👍
vitamin B12	>👍👍👍👍
calcium	>👍👍👍👍
protein	>👍👍👍👍
phosphorus	>👍👍👍👍
selenium	>👍👍👍👍
sodium	>👍👍👍👍
chloride	>👍👍👍👍
vitamin C	👍👍👍👍
niacin	👍👍👍👍
vitamin A total retinol equivalents)	👍👍👍
copper	👍👍👍
zinc	👍👍👍
folate	👍👍
riboflavin	👍👍
fibre (non-starch polysaccaride)	👍👍
iron	👍👍
magnesium	👍👍
potassium	👍👍
vitamin D	👍
thiamin	👍
iodine	👍

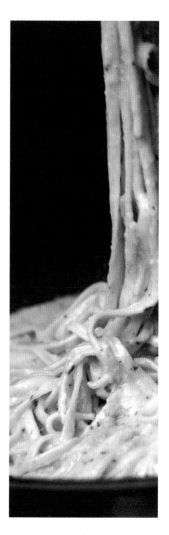

crab claw linguini with french beans & broad bean pesto

serves 4

This is definitely a dish to eat with your eyes. Use Alaskan king or spider crab for big chunks of meaty texture.

4 crab legs, approximately 80g

4 crab claws, approximately 200g

handful of fine french beans

400g dry linguini

200g broad beans

small bunch basil leaves

1 large garlic clove, crushed

150g parmesan cheese, grated, plus extra to serve

100ml olive oil

salt & pepper

To prepare the pesto cook the broad beans in boiling water for about 4-5 minutes, about half the time if using frozen. Shell and discard the skins. Next put the beans, basil, garlic and parmesan into a food processor and whiz until combined but not completely smooth. With the motor running, add the oil in a steady stream until you have a thick sauce. Season to taste.

Next steam the french beans until fully cooked then julienne them to a fine spaghetti and set aside.

Boil the pasta to al dente*. Drain, rinse well and set aside.

To prepare the crab, break the legs into sections and split the shells. Also split the underside of the claws. Prepare a pot of boiling water with a steamer. Place the crab in the steamer for approximately 5 minutes. The meat is fully cooked when it turns bright orange and opaque white. Remove the meat from shells keeping it in large chunks. It is up to you whether to remove the claw meat as well.

Warm a skillet with olive oil and toss the pasta and pesto to warm. Add parmesan, french beans and crab meat. Serve immediately.

Each portion provides 22g protein and 650kcals

*see *the basics*, page 280

nutrient	thumbs-up score
vitamin B6	👍👍👍
copper	👍👍👍
phosphorus	👍👍👍
selenium	👍👍
vitamin C	👍
folate	👍
niacin	👍
riboflavin	👍
thiamin	👍
fibre (non-starch polysaccaride)	👍
iron	👍
magnesium	👍
protein	👍
sodium	👍
chloride	👍
zinc	👍

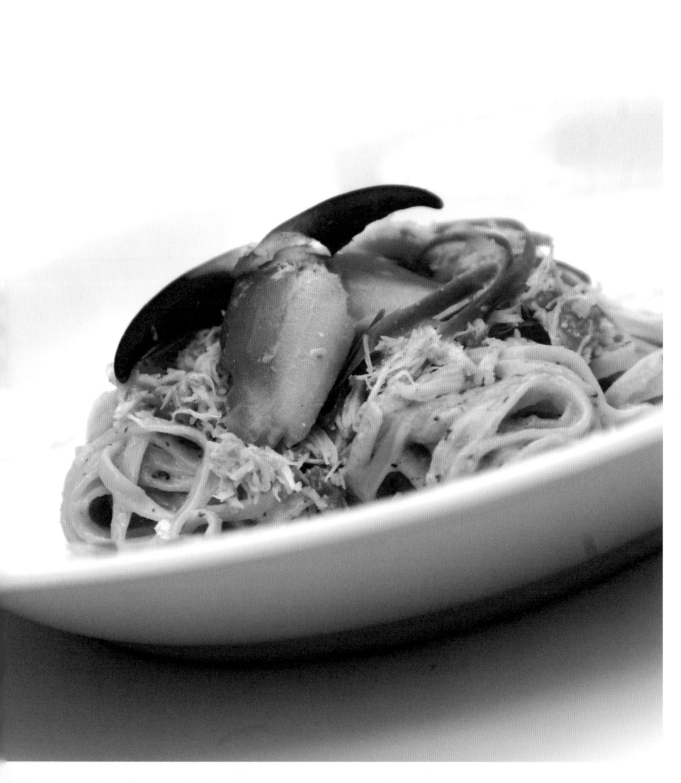

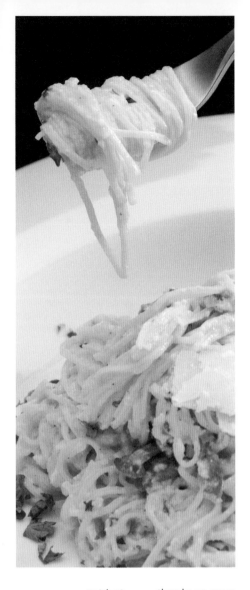

spaghetti carbonara

serves 4

This original Sardinian classic is so simple, fast and packed with goodness. The flavours are strong enough to cut through plastic or metal mouth and its creaminess is easy on the tummy.

300g spaghetti

20ml olive oil

2 garlic cloves, puréed

dash of sriracha

175g speck or lardons, diced in small cubes

5 eggs

120ml cream

100g parmesan cheese, finely grated

handful of fresh parsley, finely chopped

salt & pepper

Cook the spaghetti to al dente* in salted water. Rinse thoroughly and set aside.

Next, coat a large frying pan with a fine film of olive oil and heat the garlic and sriracha. Add the speck and simmer until cooked. Take care not to burn the garlic. Then in a separate bowl, beat the eggs and cream together.

Over a medium-low heat, add the spaghetti to the frying pan and pour in the egg mixture, tossing constantly with tongs. Add about half the cheese and keep tossing until the eggs are fully cooked. Sprinkle over the remaining cheese and garnish with parsley. Serve immediately.

Each portion provides 39g protein and 770kcals

*see *the basics*, page 280

nutrient	thumbs-up score
vitamin B12	>👍👍👍👍
phosphorus	>👍👍👍👍
sodium	>👍👍👍👍
chloride	👍👍👍👍
vitamin B6	👍👍👍
protein	👍👍👍
vitamin A (total retinol equivalents)	👍👍
riboflavin	👍👍
thiamin	👍👍
calcium	👍👍
copper	👍👍
zinc	👍👍
niacin	👍
folate	👍
iron	👍
magnesium	👍
selenium	👍

wild mushroom pappardelle in truffle cream

serves 4

This is a meal packed with flavour and soft textures. Although the mushrooms are cooked, all the juices remain in the dish.

400g egg papardelle

450g assorted wild mushrooms, trimmed & washed

black truffles optional

3 tbsp olive oil

1 garlic clove, finely diced

1 dried chilli, chopped

20ml white wine

juice of ½ lemon

knob of butter

250g parmesan, grated and extra to slice for garnish

small bunch flat parsley, coarsely chopped

300ml double cream

2-3 tbsp truffle paste

salt & pepper

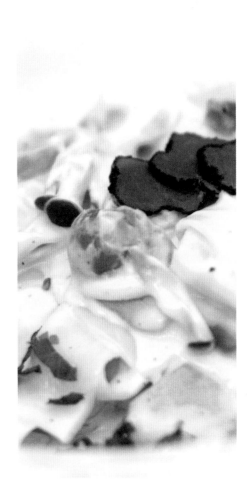

Warm butter and oil in a skillet and add mushrooms, garlic and chilli. When the pan is quite hot squeeze lemon and add a bit of wine. Toss frequently and season with a bit of salt and pepper. When mushrooms are fully cooked remove from heat.

In a saucepan add cream, truffle paste and a touch of garlic. When the cream is ready to boil add parmesan a bit at a time until cheese is fully melted. Stir constantly and do not allow to over boil. Add a knob of butter and season to taste.

Boil papardelle in salted water until al dente* then drain and rinse well. To serve, warm pasta in the sauce, top with mushrooms and parsley. Serve hot.

If wild mushrooms are not available use chestnut or small portobello. Reconstituted dried cepes also add rich strong flavour. For added texture, flavour and drama top with finely sliced black truffles.

Each portion provides 38 g protein and 1085kcals

*see *the basics*, page 280

nutrient	thumbs-up score
vitamin A (total retinol equivalents)	>👍👍👍👍
vitamin B12	>👍👍👍👍
calcium	>👍👍👍👍
copper	>👍👍👍👍
phosphorus	>👍👍👍👍
iodine	👍👍👍👍
riboflavin	👍👍👍
iron	👍👍👍
protein	👍👍👍
vitamin B6	👍👍
selenium	👍👍
zinc	👍👍
folate	👍
niacin	👍
thiamin	👍
magnesium	👍
potassium	👍
sodium	👍
chloride	👍

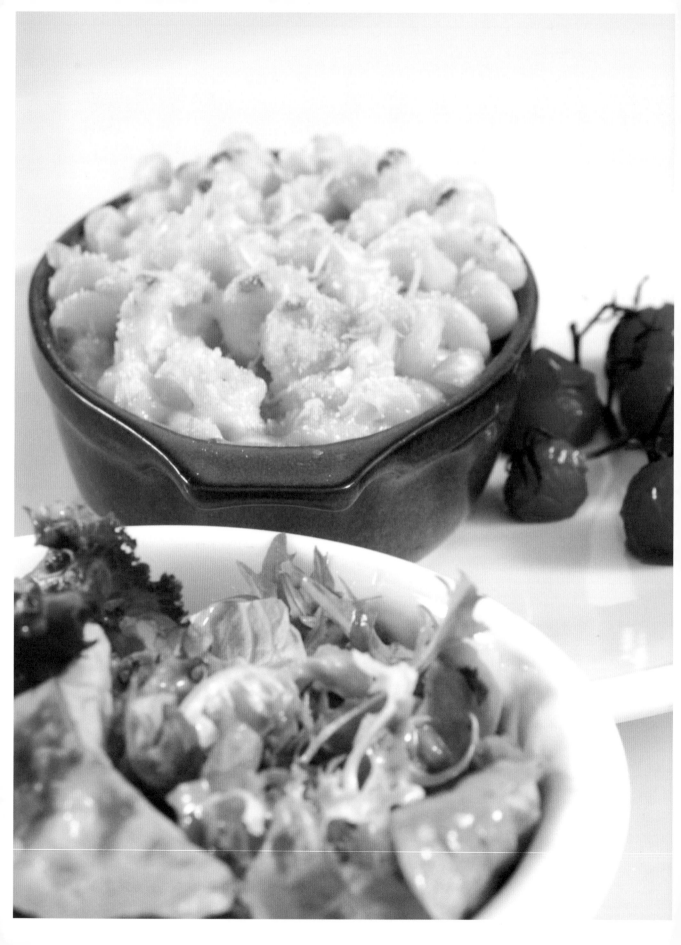

dijon & four cheese macaroni
serves 4

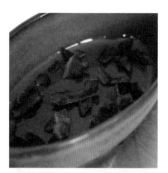

*Whenever I can't think of what to prepare I revert to 'mac 'n cheese'.
There really is nothing quite like it.*

6-8 smoked bacon rashers

250g macaroni

knob of butter

1 tbsp flour, sifted

300ml milk

2 tbsp dijon mustard

100g mature cheddar cheese, grated

50g emmenthal cheese, grated

1 tbsp cream cheese

50g parmesan cheese, grated

$1/_8$ cup breadcrumbs

salt & pepper

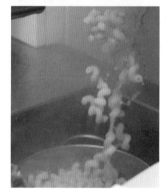

Preheat oven to 180°Cf.

Fry or grill the bacon until crisp then pat dry and break into pieces.
Cook the macaroni thoroughly; you do not want the pasta al dente
as it will absorb the cheese sauce when baking.

To make the cheese sauce, start by making a roux* and gently
warming the milk. Gradually add the warmed milk to the roux,
stirring constantly. Lightly season and add the mustard. Cook but
don't boil for about 2 minutes. Never stop stirring!

Gradually add the cream cheese and cheese in small amounts
melting thoroughly. Keep tasting as the sauce thickens adjust
seasoning as required. Leave on a gentle boil for several minutes
until reduced by one third. Finally, stir in a knob of butter.

Butter a casserole dish. Add the bacon and cooked macaroni.
Cover with the cheese sauce then sprinkle with parmesan and
breadcrumbs. Bake for 20 minutes or until the top is golden brown.

Each portion provides 39g protein and 740kcals

*see *the basics*, page 282

nutrient	thumbs-up score
vitamin B6	>👍👍👍👍
sodium	👍👍👍
chloride	👍👍👍
vitamin C	👍
thiamin	👍
calcium	👍
copper	👍
fibre (as non-starch polysaccharide)	👍
folate	👍
iron	👍
phosphorus	👍
protein	👍

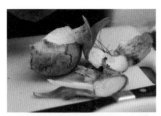

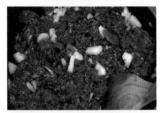

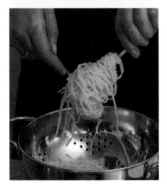

angel hair ragu

serves 4

This is comfort on every level and packed with goodness. The flavours are strong enough to tackle plastic or metal mouth.

55g butter
drizzle olive oil
2-3 garlic cloves, crushed
1 large carrot, finely chopped
1 stalk celery, finely chopped
1 medium onion, finely chopped
55g minced pancetta
100g minced lean beef
100g minced lean pork
dash of sriracha
800g chopped tomatoes, 2 tins
1 glass of red wine
a little beef or chicken stock
3 tbsp tomato purée
handful of dried italian herbs
salt & pepper
500g fresh or 400g dried egg angel hair or spaghettini
60g parmesan cheese, grated

Heat the oil and butter in a large pan, add 1 clove garlic, carrot, celery and onion and cook without colour, about 10 minutes on low heat. Add the tomatoes and half the herbs and cook for another 30 minutes seasoning to taste. Liquidise the mixture.

In a lightly oiled pan, brown the pancetta and minced meats with remaining garlic, sriracha, herbs and seasoning. When browned, add wine and stir in a little stock. Next add tomato purée and dilute with a bit more stock as required. Place the tomato mixture and meat in a pot and simmer for approximately 1½ hours, adding stock as the sauce reduces. Season to taste.

Cook the pasta in boiling salted water until al dente.* Drain and rinse well and mix with the sauce. Serve with parmesan cheese.

Each portion provides 37g protein and 700kcals

*see *the basics*, page 280

nutrient	thumbs-up score
vitamin A (total retinol equivalents	>👍👍👍👍
vitamin B6	>👍👍👍👍
copper	>👍👍👍👍
phosphorus	👍👍👍👍
vitamin B12	👍👍👍
iodine	👍👍👍
protein	👍👍👍
sodium	👍👍👍
chloride	👍👍👍
vitamin C	👍👍
thiamin	👍👍
calcium	👍👍
iron	👍👍
selenium	👍👍
zinc	👍👍
riboflavin	👍
niacin	👍
fibre (as non-starch polysaccharide)	👍
folate	👍
magnesium	👍
potassium	👍

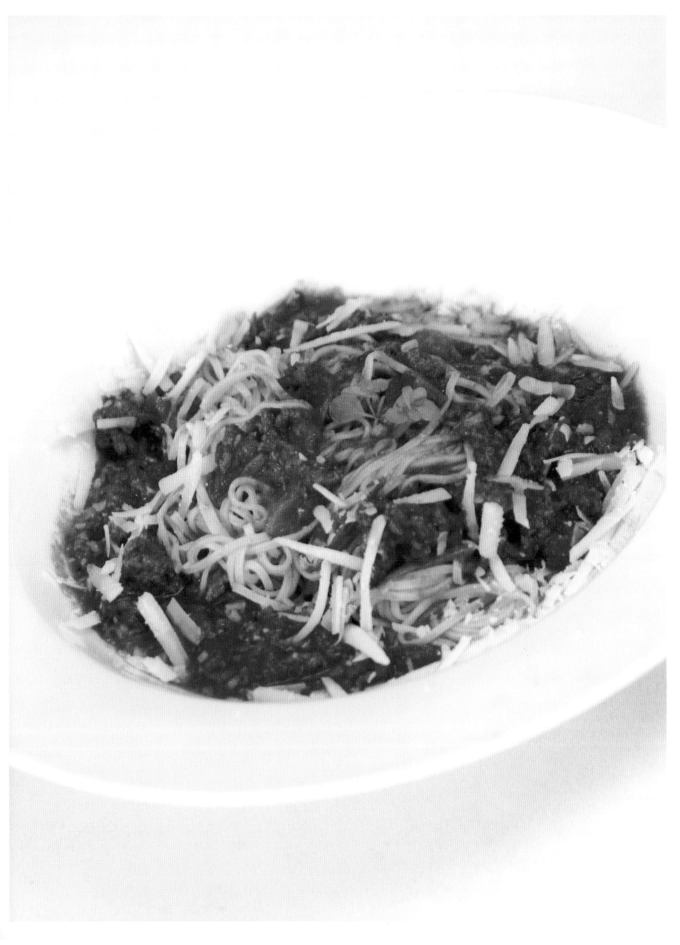

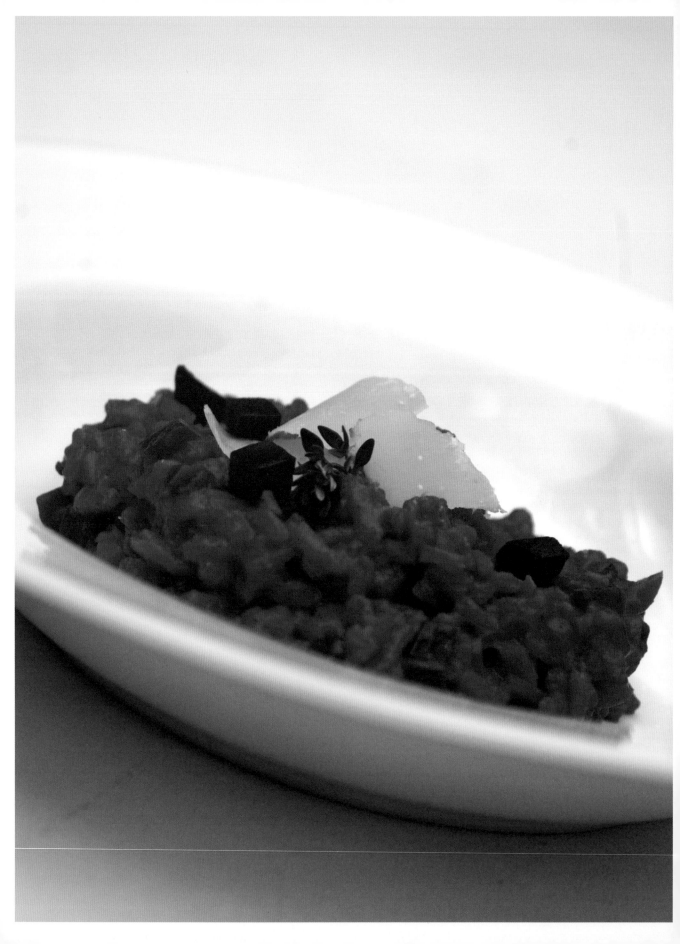

creamy beetroot risotto

serves 4

The colour of this is simply marvellous. It's wonderful as a dish on its own and a great partner with fish and shellfish. I love it with langoustine.

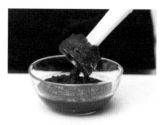

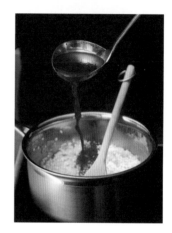

500g beetroot
2 tbsp olive oil
1 onion, finely diced
1 garlic clove, puréed
250g risotto rice
150ml white wine
700ml vegetable stock
salt & pepper
a few shavings parmesan
a few sprigs of fresh dill
crème fraiche

Preheat oven to 180°Cf.

Cut the beetroot into quarters, lightly brush with oil and place in the oven on a baking tray. Roast for 1 hour or until soft. Set aside to cool then remove the skins. Purée half with a hand blender and finely dice the other half.

Coat the bottom of a pan with oil, melt butter then add the onion and garlic and cook without colour on medium heat. Add the rice and stir to coat the grains and allow to warm. Pour in the wine and simmer for 1 minute.

Add the beetroot purée to the stock and start adding this to the rice a ladle at a time allowing the rice to absorb the stock and checking the seasoning as you go. When the rice is al dente stir in the beetroot and a bit of the cheese. Season to taste. Garnish with a dollop of crème fraiche, a few shavings of parmesan and a sprinkle of dill. Serve immediately.

Each portion provides 10g protein and 360kcals

nutrient	thumbs-up score
sodium	👍👍👍
chloride	👍👍
folate	👍👍
phosphorus	👍👍
vitamin B6	👍
thiamin	👍
calcium	👍
copper	👍
fibre (non-starch polysaccaride)	👍
potassium	👍
protein	👍
zinc	👍

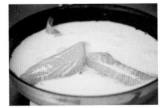

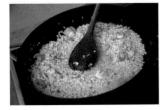

smoked haddock with pea & baby leek risotto

serves 4

This risotto is packed with flavour, texture and nutrition. It might look a bit fiddly but it's quite straight forward and what a result!

1 large shallot, finely chopped

1 small leek, white only finely sliced

1 bay leaf

sprig of thyme

splash of olive oil

large knob of butter

225g risotto rice

150ml white wine

500ml vegetable stock

small handful of parsley, finely chopped

50g petit pois

500ml milk

1 filet smoked haddock, undyed

juice of ½ lemon

20g cream cheese

4 organic free-range eggs, optional

Place the butter, shallot, leek, bay leaf and thyme in a pan and cook without colour. Stir in the rice and coat with the mixture and allow to warm for a minute. Discard the bay leaf and thyme stalk and pour in the wine. Start adding the stock a ladle at a time allowing the rice to absorb the moisture.

In the meantime, bring the milk to a simmer in another pan. Poach the haddock for 1-2 minutes. Lift from the milk, remove the skin, break into chunks and sprinkle with lemon juice.

When the risotto is al dente stir in the cream cheese, peas and parsley and gently fold in the haddock.

Poach the eggs*. To serve spoon risotto into a shallow bowl, top with egg. Serve immediately.

Each portion provides 22g protein and 490kcals

*see *the basics*, page 282

nutrient	thumbs-up score
vitamin B12	>👍👍👍👍
iodine	>👍👍👍👍
phosphorus	👍👍👍
vitamin B6	👍👍
riboflavin	👍👍
protein	👍👍
sodium	👍👍
chloride	👍
vitamin A total retinol equivalents)	👍
folate	👍
niacin	👍
thiamin	👍
calcium	👍
copper	👍
selenium	👍
zinc	👍

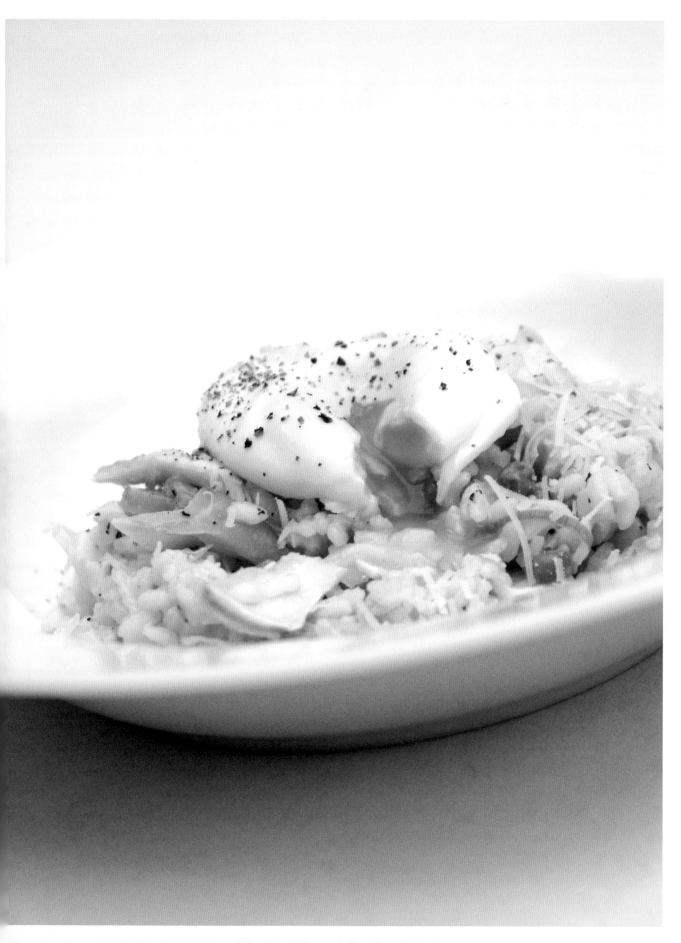

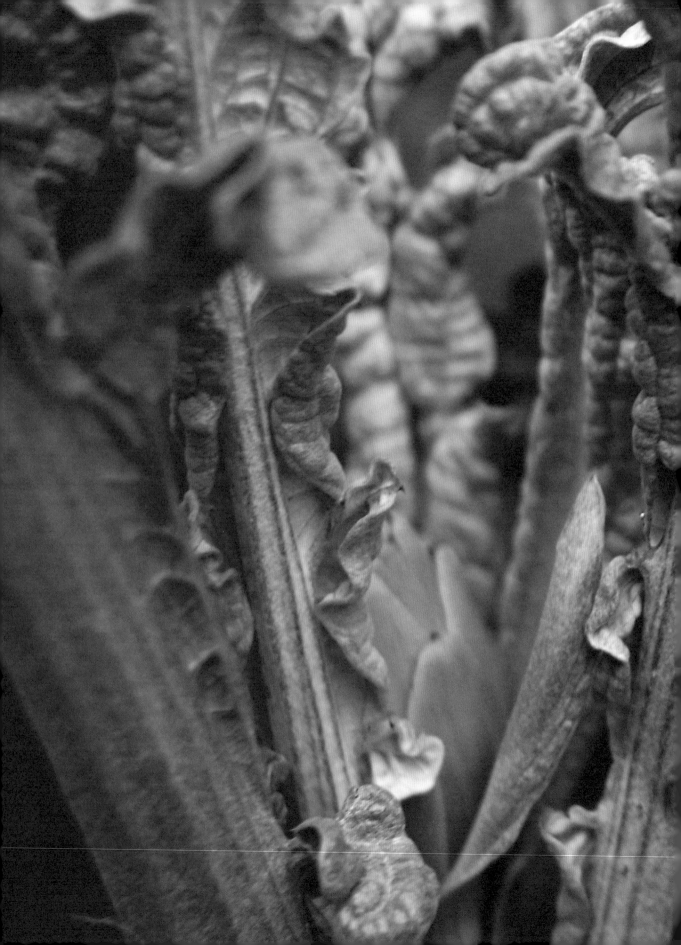

vegetables
& side dishes

vegetables & side dishes

potato dauphinoise	148
refried pinto beans	150
puy lentils & shallots	151
swede & potato mash	153
onions roasted with ginger	153
roasted okra	154
stuffed globe courgette	155
asparagus wrapped in prosciutto with melon	156
globe artichokes with lemon mayo	158
creamy cheesy leeks	159
sauté of asian vegetables	161
jasmine coconut rice	162
french petit pois & pearl onions	162
mushroom duxelle	164
french beans & onion ring casserole	165
broccoli purée	166
brittany courgette	167
potato rosti	168
potato purée	170
simply the best yorkshire pudding	171
shallot tart	173

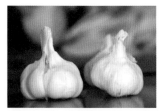

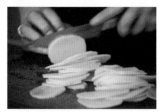

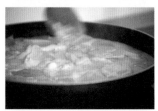

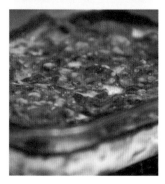

potato dauphinoise
serves 4

These potatoes are simply the best! So rich and creamy and the aroma is like no other. If waking up the tastebuds was an Olympic sport, potatoes dauphinoise would take the gold medal!

7-8 waxy potatoes
3 garlic cloves, crushed
dash of sriracha
splash of olive oil
200ml double cream
200g crème fraiche
120g parmesan cheese, finely grated
300ml milk
salt & white pepper

Preheat oven to 170°Cf.

Peel potatoes and slice finely with a mandolin or sharp knife.

In a lightly oiled, deep frying pan, heat the garlic and sriracha. Pour in a little cream, then layers of potatoes separated by equal pouring of double cream and crème fraiche and sprinkles of parmesan and pepper. Fill the pan with milk and simmer for about 15 minutes until really starchy.

Transfer the potatoes to a buttered baking dish. Add more milk if the mixture seems a bit dry. Cover with parmesan, salt and pepper. Bake for 1-1½ hours until the potatoes are soft to a sharp knife and the surface is nicely golden. Leave for at least 20 minutes before serving.

This dish can be prepared the night before and then cut with a scone cutter to make elegant little towers.

Each portion provides 18g protein and 690kcals

nutrient	thumbs-up score
vitamin A (total retinol equivalents)	>👍👍👍👍
vitamin B6	>👍👍👍👍
vitamin B12	>👍👍👍👍
calcium	👍👍👍
phosphorous	👍👍👍
iodine	👍👍
sodium	👍👍
chloride	👍👍
vitamin C	👍
riboflavin	👍
copper	👍
potassium	👍
protein	👍
zinc	👍

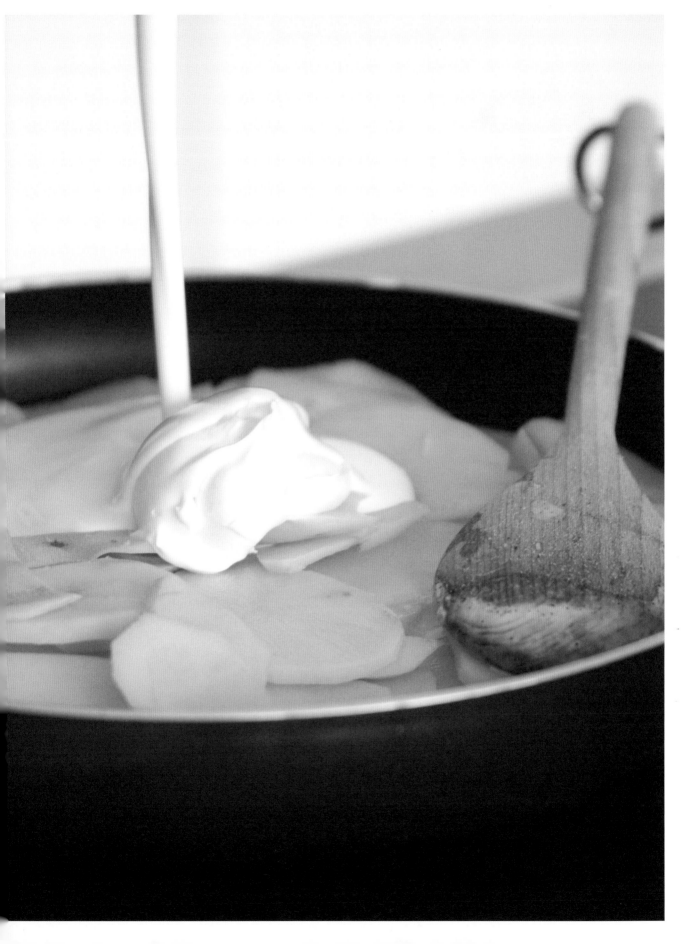

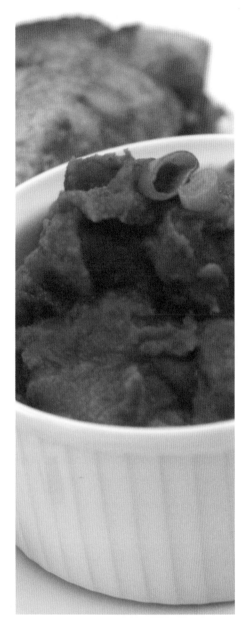

refried pinto beans
serves 4-6 as a side

Unsurprisingly these are best served with chicken enchiladas, tacos, salsa and maybe a margarita. They are soft and mild so easy to eat and digest.

200g dried pinto beans, (or half pinto and half black beans)
2 bay leaves
1 whole bulb garlic
175ml olive oil
1 tin chopped tomatoes
3 tsp salt
1 cup spring onions, chopped

Rinse the beans thoroughly. Discard any that are shriveled. Place in a pan with 8 cups water. Do not add any salt as this can dry out the beans. Add the bay leaves and bring to the boil, then lower the heat and simmer for 2 hours or until the beans are soft. Add more boiling water as required to keep the level up and stir occasionally.

Preheat oven to 200°Cf

Brush the garlic bulb with oil and roast for 15-20 minutes. The flesh should squeeze easily from the husks. Remove any excess water from the beans and add the rest of the oil, tomatoes, garlic and salt. Allow to simmer for another 1½ hours. Don't rush this, as you want the flavours to intensify and the texture to soften. When soft, lightly mash and season to taste. Sprinkle over the chopped spring onion and serve warm.

Each portion provides 8g protein and 110kcals

nutrient	thumbs-up score
sodium	👍👍👍👍
chloride	👍👍👍👍
folate	👍👍
vitamin B6	👍
vitamin C	👍
thiamin	👍
copper	👍
fibre (non-starch polysaccaride)	👍
iron	👍
phosphorus	👍
potassium	👍

puy lentils & shallots
serves 4-6 as a side

Protein rich puy lentils come from France and are unique for their peppery flavour. They also hold their texture nicely so are great served as a side dish. Perfect with lamb and game.

300g puy lentils
1 cube vegetable stock
splash of olive oil
1 knob of butter
dash of sriracha
2 large shallots, finely chopped
2 sticks celery, finely chopped
1 tbsp rosemary, chopped
1 tbsp marjoram, chopped
2 tbsp parsley, chopped
salt & pepper

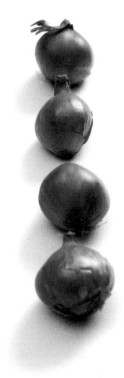

Put the lentils and stock cube in a pan with lots of water and bring to the boil then cover and simmer for 20 minutes or until the lentils are cooked al dente. Remove them from the heat but leave them in the stock.

Melt the butter in a lightly oiled pan and cook the shallots with a bit of colour. Remove from heat and mix in the herbs.

Make sure the lentils are cooked through, they should be soft but hold their shape. Drain and return to the pan. Stir in the shallots. Season to taste and serve hot or cold.

Each portion provides 19g protein and 260kcals

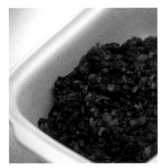

nutrient	thumbs-up score
selenium	>👍👍👍👍
iron	👍👍👍👍
vitamin B6	👍👍👍
copper	👍👍👍
phosphorus	👍👍
sodium	👍👍
chloride	👍👍
folate	👍
thiamin	👍
fibre (non-starch polysaccharide)	👍
magnesium	👍
potassium	👍
protein	👍
zinc	👍

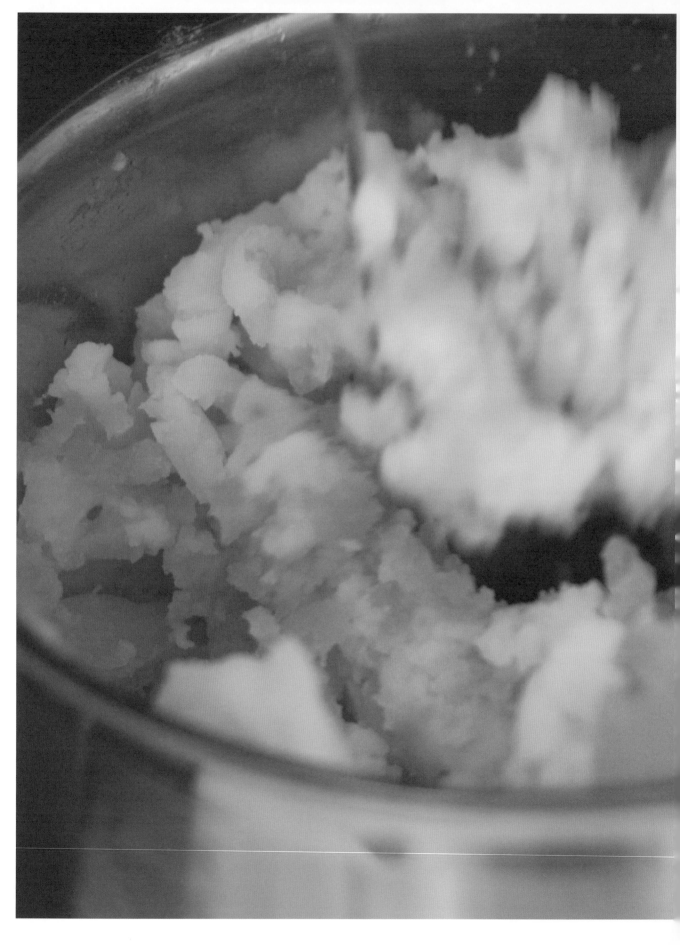

swede & potato mash

serves 4

This is a simple way to add a bit of variety, colour and stronger flavour to ordinary mash. For added nutritional value, whip in an egg. It's great with lamb.

350g floury potatoes
350g swede
120ml milk
50g butter
white pepper

Peel and cut equal amounts of potato and swede. Boil until soft, then pass through a ricer for a smooth purée or mash for a courser texture. Add milk, butter and white pepper to taste.

Each portion provides 3g protein and 150kcals

nutrient	thumbs-up score
vitamin B6	>👍👍👍👍
vitamin C	👍👍
vitamin A (total retinol equivalents)	👍
vitamin B12	👍

onions roasted with ginger

serves 4

On its own a single onion doesn't deliver a huge amount of nutritional value but it makes a great contribution to flavour for meat and vegetable dishes alike.

4 small cooking onions
3cm ginger, fine julienne
olive oil

Preheat oven to 160°Cf.

Trim and peel the onions then remove the very centre (the end of a chopstick works well for this). Stuff 3-4 slivers of ginger into the onions then coat with a fine film of oil and place in a roasting dish and into the oven. Roast until cooked through but still firm and golden brown. If the outer layer of the onion gets a bit crispy, peel it off. Serve hot.

Each portion provides 1g protein and 24kcals

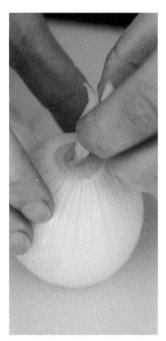

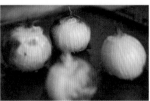

nutrient	thumbs-up score

The nutritional analysis measures lower than 20% RNI due to small portion size.

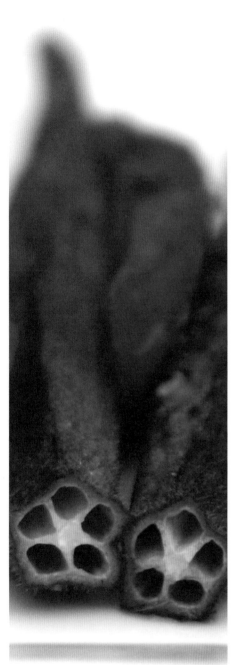

roasted okra
serves 4

I included these because many people look at these beauties at the market but don't know a basic preparation and they are a perfect curry and creole partner. So here's a really simple method.

20 okra
2 italian tomatoes, seeded and cut into fine petals
drizzle of olive oil
salt & pepper

Preheat oven to 180°Cf.

Line a baking pan with tin foil. Trim the tops off and place the okra and tomatoes petals flat on the tray. Drizzle with oil and season. Roast for 12-15 minutes or until the okra is cooked through. That's it! Serve hot.

Simply roasting the vegetables keeps them from becoming too gummy as well.

Each portion provides 2g protein and 25kcals

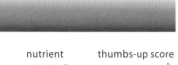

nutrient	thumbs-up score
vitamin C	👍
sodium	👍
chloride	👍

stuffed globe courgette

serves 4

This is a small portion veggie take on stuffed marrow. If you can't get globe courgette use large regular ones by splitting down the middle like mini marrows. They're fab.

4 globe courgette
splash of olive oil
1 onion, finely chopped
2 large shallots, finely chopped
4 italian tomatoes, de-seeded and finely chopped
1 garlic clove, puréed
2 tbsp flat parsley, chopped
leaves from 1 sprig of thyme
50ml white wine
40g parmesan cheese, grated
salt & pepper

Cut the tops off the courgettes, set them aside and scoop out the seeds and string and discard then scoop out some of the flesh so that the cavity is about an inch thick. Roughly chop the flesh.

In an oiled pan, cook the onions and shallots without colour then add the courgette flesh, tomatoes, garlic, parsley, thyme and wine. Allow to cook until excess moisture has evaporated stirring gently from time to time. Season to taste.

Preheat oven to 180°Cf.

When ready to stuff and bake, mix in most of the cheese, leaving a little for the top of each. Stuff the cavities to slightly over full then sprinkle on the remaining cheese and replace the tops as little hats. The cheese will act as glue to keep them in place. Place on a baking tray in the oven for about 30-40 minutes. You know they are done when you give them a light squeeze and they give but are still firm.

Each portion provides 7g protein and 100kcals

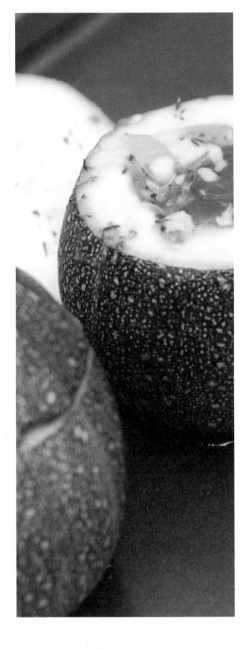

nutrient	thumbs-up score
vitamin C	👍👍
vitamin A (total retinol equivalents)	👍
vitamin B6	👍
vitamin B12	👍
folate	👍
calcium	👍
phosphorus	👍
potassium	👍
sodium	👍
chloride	👍

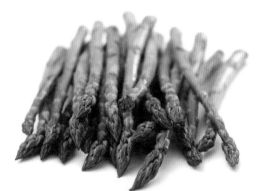

asparagus wrapped in prosciutto with melon

serves 4, 2 parcels per person

This is such a quick and fun way to serve asparagus. The melon is a soothing texture for dry mouth and a sore throat.

12 spears large asparagus
4-6 slices prosciutto
1 ripe cantelope melon

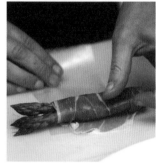

Break the asparagus ends off and trim so you are left with the tender green spears and tops. Lightly steam until cooked through yet still firm.

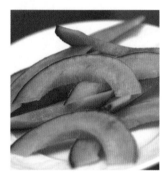

Wrap two or three together in a slice of prosciutto and serve with sliced melon. Easy!

Each portion provides 8g protein and 65kcals

nutrient	thumbs-up score
vitamin C	👍
sodium	👍

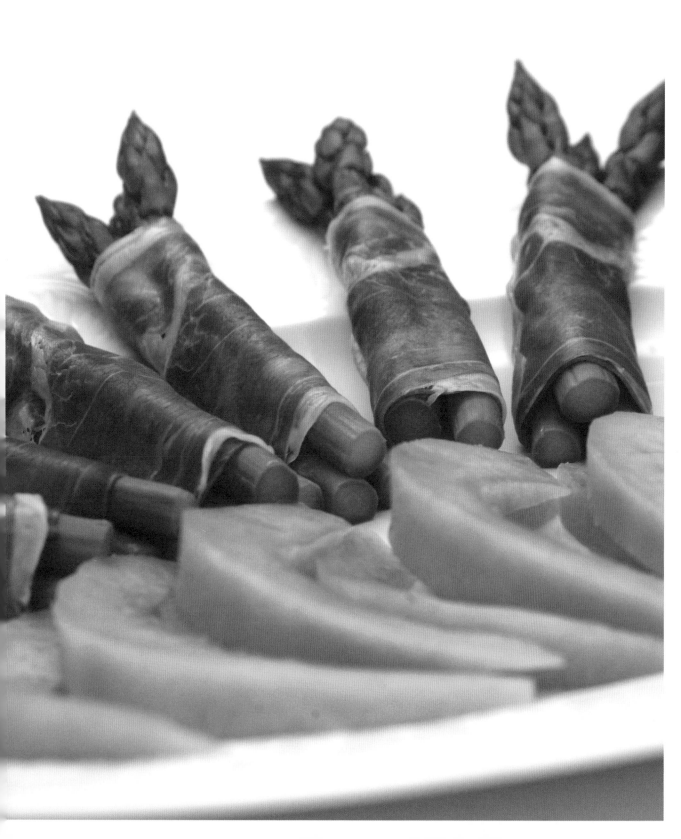

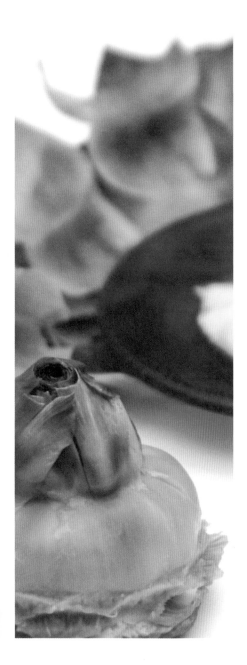

globe artichokes with lemon mayo
serves 4

These are simply my favourite. It takes awhile to work through all the leaves and getting to the heart is a bit of a pfaff but it's worth it. Go the extra mile and make fresh mayonnaise.

4 large globe artichokes
400g lemon mayonnaise* (about ¼ cup per serving)
1 lemon, cut into 4 wedges

Put a pan of water large enough to hold and submerge the artichokes on high heat and bring to the boil.

Top and tail the artichokes by cutting about 1 inch off the top of the leaves and cut the stem off just into the leaves. Remove any small and very tough leaves from the bottom. Fully submerge the artichokes in the water, turn down the heat and allow to simmer for 30-40 minutes. Check them frequently as the time will vary due to size. They are done when the base is soft but firm and a knife will slide into the heart at the bottom. Don't overcook. Drain the artichokes on paper towel to remove excess moisture and remove any loose leaves from the bottom.

Make the mayonnaise*. If using store-bought, squeeze in some lemon juice to give it some zing.

Serve with mayonnaise on the side and a bowl for discarding the leaves. Tear off each leaf and dip in the mayonnaise, eating only the tender inside flesh. When you get to the thin leaves and 'hair' inside, use a knife or spoon to lift this away and discard leaving the lovely round heart as your reward.

Each portion provides 5g protein and 800kcals

*see *the basics*, page 284

nutrient	thumbs-up score
vitamin B12	👍👍👍
folate	👍👍👍
sodium	👍
chloride	👍

creamy cheesy leeks

serves 4 as a side

Leeks are so full of flavour and are true nutritional best friends. They are great with roast chicken or turkey.

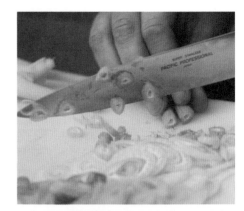

2 leeks, white only, sliced
2 shallots, peeled and finely chopped
splash of olive oil
40g butter
2 sprigs thyme
75ml white wine
120ml double cream
salt & pepper
50g gruyere cheese, finely grated

Melt butter in a lightly oiled pan. Add the leeks, shallots and thyme and cook without colour. Lightly season and add white wine. Sauté on low heat for another 2 minutes then add the cream and continue to cook until the mixture is thickening but not dry.

Preheat oven to 180°Cf.

Transfer the leeks into a greased casserole, cover with cheese and bake until the cheese is melted and light golden. Serve hot.

Each portion provides 4g protein and 290kcals

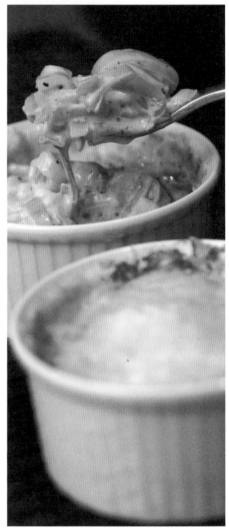

nutrient	thumbs-up score
vitamin A (total retinol equivalents)	👍👍
sodium	👍👍
chloride	👍👍
vitamin B12	👍
calcium	👍

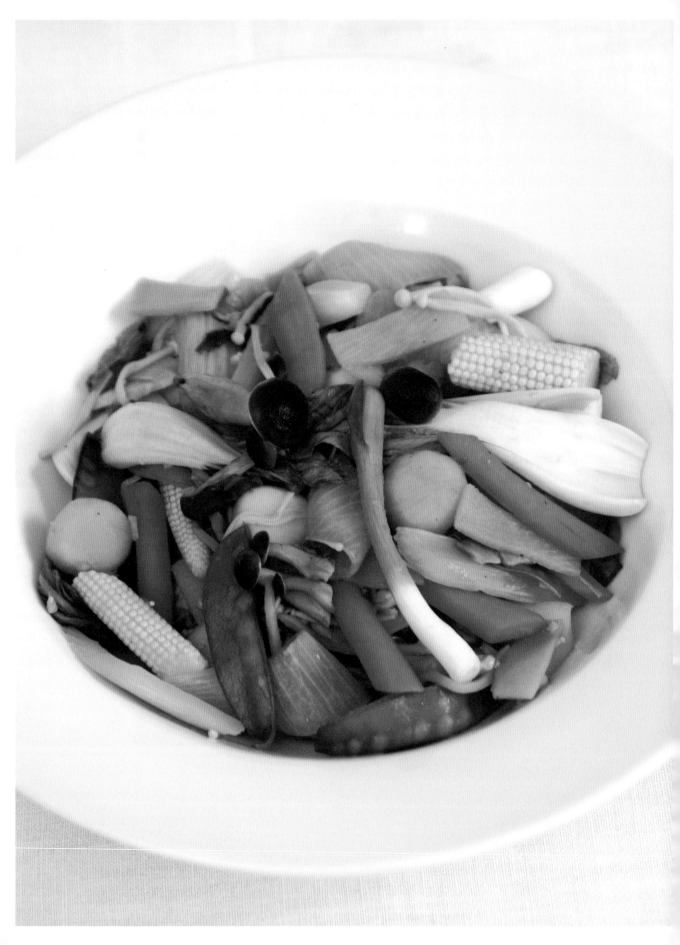

sauté of asian vegetables
serves 4

These are such fresh and flavourful vegetables. The stir-fry keeps all the water-soluble vitamins in. They're a perfect accompliment to fish like tuna. Mmm!

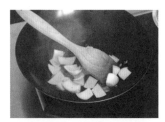

1 tbsp ground nut oil
1 garlic clove, puréed
dash of sriracha
150g baby corn
1 thai green pepper, chopped
150g baby pak choi, chopped
150g shitake mushrooms
1 onion, quartered
2 celery stalks, cut into 2 inch sticks
150g small whole green onions
1 tbsp tamari soy sauce
3cm fresh ginger, peeled and finely julienned
1 tbsp mirin

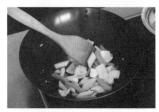

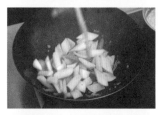

Warm the garlic and oil in a wok. Add the sriracha and vegetables and stir-fry for a minute or two, then add the soy sauce, ginger and mirin. Simmer until just cooked through. Serve hot in a big bowl with the juices.

Each portion provides 3g protein and 95kcals

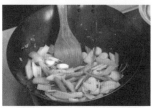

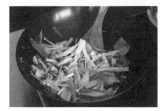

nutrient	thumbs-up score
vitamin C	👍👍
sodium	👍👍
chloride	👍👍
vitamin B6	👍

nutrient	thumbs-up score
copper	👍
phosphorus	👍

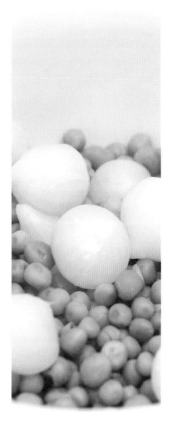

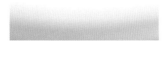

nutrient	thumbs-up score
fibre (non-starch polysaccaride)	👍👍
phosphorus	👍👍
vitamin A (total retinol equivalents)	👍
vitamin C	👍
vitamin B6	👍
folate	👍
thiamin	👍
copper	👍
iron	👍
protein	👍
sodium	👍
zinc	👍

jasmine coconut rice

serves 4

This rice is lovely with fish and curries.

1 cup jasmine rice
1 cup water
1 cup coconut milk

Cook the rice in the water with coconut milk. Bring just to the boil then turn heat to low and allow the rice to absorb the liquid. When nearly cooked turn the heat off and be careful not to burn the bottom of the pan. Serve hot.

Each portion provides 5g protein and 250kcals

french petit pois & pearl onions

serves 4

These dressed up peas pack in extra nutrition and flavour.

750g petit pois, frozen
small splash of olive oil
large knob of butter
200g white pearl onions, blanched and skinned
3 rashers streaky, smoked bacon, cut into lardons
1 garlic clove, finely chopped
½ small loose leaf lettuce, finely shredded
¼ cube chicken stock
1 tsp thyme leaves
¼ cup water, as needed

Thaw the peas on paper towel. Melt oil and butter together then add the bacon and onion for 2-3 minutes. Stir in the garlic, lettuce, stock cube and thyme and season with a bit of pepper. Next add the peas with a small amount of water and simmer on low heat for 5 minutes stirring occasionally and adding just enough moisture if the mixture gets dry. Serve in a large bowl and top with butter.

Each portion provides 14g protein and 200kcals

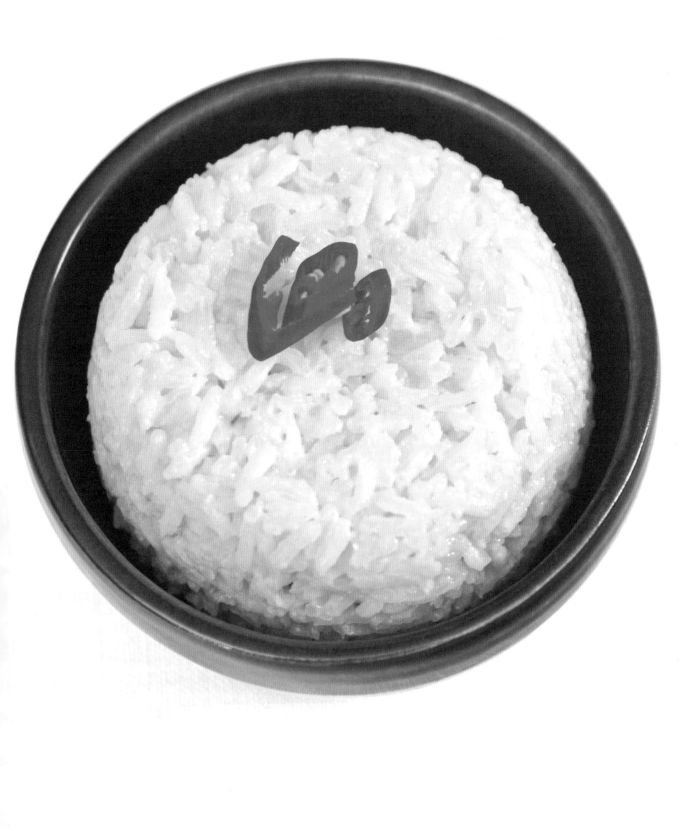

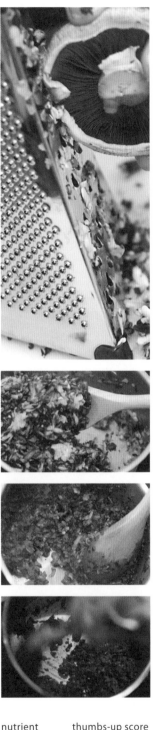

mushroom duxelle

Duxelle has been a staple since the 17th century. Although best known for it's contribution to Beef Wellington, it's a fabulous partner for so many dishes.

4 large shallots, finely chopped
knob of butter
dash of sriracha
200g mushrooms, finely chopped
1 tbsp dijon mustard
salt & pepper

The shallots and mushrooms are best prepared with a food processor or cheese grater.

Sauté the shallots in butter until soft and without colour. Add the mushrooms and cook for around 30 minutes until the mixture has reduced and is quite dry. Add the mustard and sriracha and season to taste.

Each portion provides 2g protein and 35kcals

nutrient	thumbs-up score
copper	👍
sodium	👍
chloride	👍

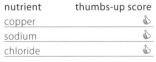

french bean & onion ring casserole
serves 4-6 as a side

This is vintage American comfort food at its finest. It never seems to grow tired. It's so morish so no wonder!

900g french beans, trimmed

50g butter

splash of olive oil

1 onion, chopped

225g button or small cup mushrooms, sliced

1 garlic clove, finely chopped

leaves of 2 thyme sprigs

2 tbsp flour

150ml white wine

250ml vegetable stock

120ml double cream

salt & pepper

225g gruyere, finely grated

handful of fine breadcrumbs

½ cup fried onion rings*, coarsely chopped

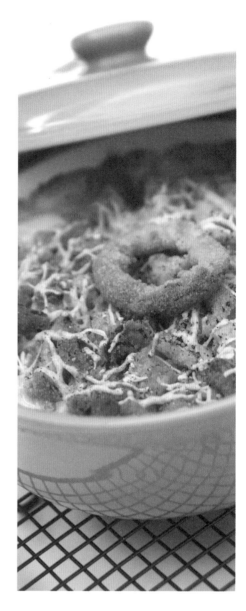

*Use store-bought frozen onion rings and follow the package instructions to cook them so they are crispy but not burned.

Boil enough salted water to blanche the beans. When they have softened plunge them in cold water, drain and set aside to dry.

Melt a knob of butter on medium-low heat in a lightly oiled pan and cook the onions without colour. Add the mushrooms, garlic and thyme and sauté for 10 minutes allowing the mushrooms to slightly caramelise then sprinkle on flour and mix. Stir in the wine, stock and cream and allow the mixture to thicken. Add extra stock if it gets too thick. Finally stir in the beans and cheese.

Preheat oven to 180°Cf.

Transfer the mixture to a greased casserole, top with onion ring pieces and sprinkle with breadcrumbs. Bake until the casserole is bubbling and golden brown on top. Serve hot.

Each portion provides 19g protein and 565kcals

nutrient	thumbs-up score
vitamin A (total retinol equivalents)	👍👍👍👍
calcium	👍👍👍👍
vitamin B12	👍👍👍
phosphorus	👍👍👍
sodium	👍👍👍
chloride	👍👍👍
copper	👍👍
vitamin B6	👍
folate	👍
riboflavin	👍
protein	👍

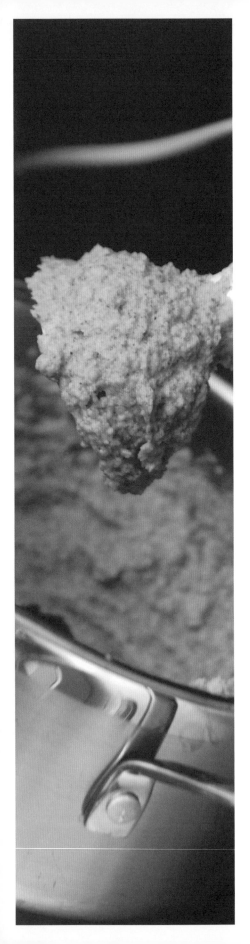

broccoli purée
serve as a side dish

I think this is a perfect accompaniment to salmon in flavour texture and colour.

800g broccoli florets
1 very small garlic clove, finely chopped
100ml olive oil
¼ tsp white pepper
salt & pepper

Cook the broccoli in boiling water until they are fully cooked but not soggy. You should be able to pierce them with a knife. Drain them well and transfer to a bowl. Add the garlic, oil, white pepper and purée with a hand mixer. Season to taste. Gently reheat before serving.

Each portion provides 9g protein and 70kcals

brittany courgette
serve as a side dish

This is just a lovely way to serve courgette. It's a nice accompaniment to roast chicken or game.

5 courgettes, diced into fine cubes
splash of olive oil
3 garlic cloves, puréed
drop of sriracha
salt & pepper

Warm garlic and sriracha in a deep oiled saucepan. Add the courgette and let stew on low heat for about 2 hours. Stir lightly with a wooden spoon so cubes do not lose their shape. Season to taste and serve as a side dish.

Each portion provides 4g protein and 37kcals

nutrient	thumbs-up score
vitamin C	>👍👍👍
folate	👍👍
vitamin A (total retinol equivalents)	👍
vitamin B6	👍
fibre (non-starch polysaccaride)	👍
phosphorus	👍
potassium	👍
sodium	👍
chloride	👍

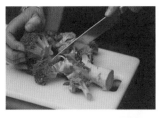

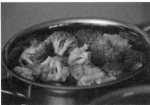

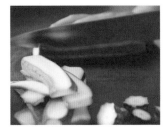

nutrient	thumbs-up score
vitamin C	👍👍
vitamin A (total retinol equivalents)	👍
vitamin B6	👍
folate	👍
potassium	👍
sodium	👍
chloride	👍
riboflavin	👍
iodine	👍

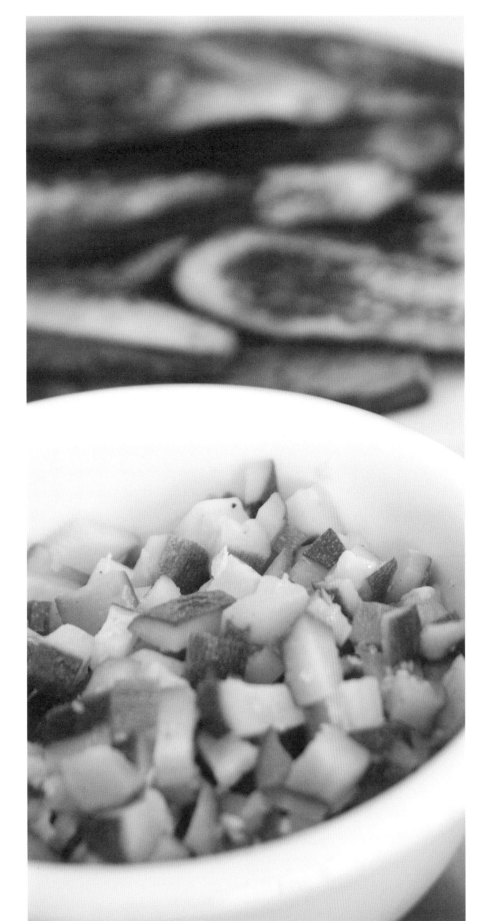

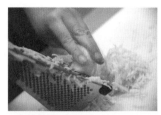

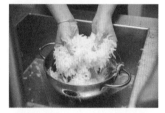

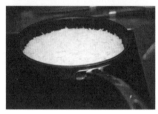

potato rosti

serves 4

Rosti is a knockout served with just about anything. It's an easy at home option to triple cooked chips. Ooh, I just love it.

1 onion, finely chopped
45g butter
1 tsp olive oil
650g waxy potatoes
salt & pepper

You need a 9 inch, non-stick frying pan for this.

Melt half the butter and oil in the pan over low heat. Cook the onions without colour and remove from the heat.

Peel and cut the potatoes into large even chunks. Place in a large saucepan, fill with cold water and lightly salt. Bring to the boil and simmer for 5 minutes. They should still be firm. Drain, dry and allow to cool slightly then coarsely grate the potatoes. Gently stir in the onions and season to taste.

Heat the remaining butter with a tiny splash of oil over low heat and add the potatoes making a flat cake with a fork. Allow to cook for 15 minutes shaking the pan frequently so the potatoes do not stick. Continue until the bottom is a golden crust.

To flip the rosti, place a plate larger than the pan on top and flip them together. Quickly slide the rosti, uncooked side down back into the pan and cook for another 15 minutes or until this side also has a golden crust. Season to taste and cut into wedges to serve.

Each portion provides 4g protein and 220kcals

nutrient	thumbs-up score
vitamin B6	👍👍👍
vitamin C	👍
vitamin D	👍
sodium	👍
chloride	👍

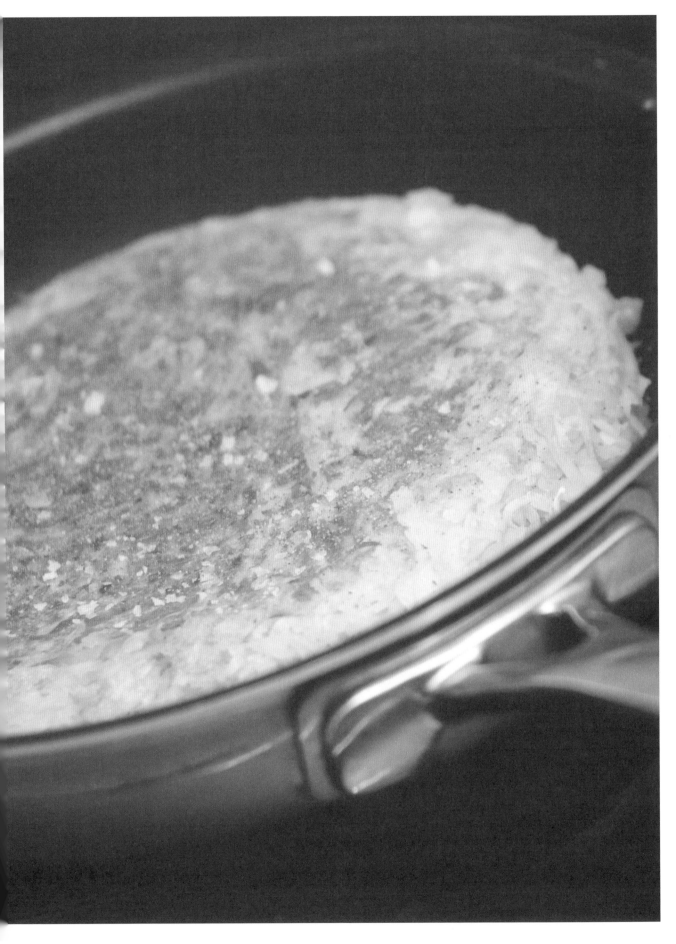

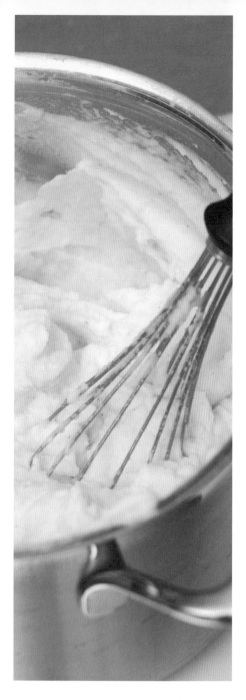

potato purée
serves 4

Potato purée is the king of all comfort foods!

675-700g floury potatoes
100ml milk
60g butter
salt & white pepper
nutmeg, freshly grated

Peel the potatoes and chop into 2-3 inch chunks. Place in a pot of cold salted water then boil until potatoes are fully cooked through. A knife or fork should pass easily through but the flesh should not fall apart.

Fully drain the potatoes then transfer to a bowl. Pass the potatoes through a ricer back into the original pot. Next, whisk in the butter and milk until the consistency is smooth and creamy but with body. Season to taste and grate in a bit of nutmeg.

A couple helpful hints with potatoes – if you can buy them from a market with the dirt still on do so. It will ensure that the potatoes have not been refrigerated so the flesh will be lovely and no nutritional value will be lost. If you don't have a ricer, break the potatoes up with a masher then finish them with a strong whisk and good-old-fashioned elbow grease. Finally, wherever possible, use the potato water for your sauces and gravies to keep the water-soluble nutrients.

Each portion provides 5g protein and 260kcals

nutrient	thumbs-up score
chloride	👍👍
sodium	👍
vitamin A (total retinol equivalents)	👍
vitamin B6	👍
vitamin B12	👍
vitamin C	👍
folate	👍
thiamin	👍
potassium	👍

simply the best yorkshire pudding

serves 4-6

I've included this recipe because it is simply the easiest and best one I've ever come across and I love them with any roast dinner.

140g plain flour
4 eggs
200ml milk
salt & pepper
splash of sunflower oil for cooking

Preheat oven to 230°Cf.

Drizzle some oil into 6-8 non-stick muffin tins or a 9x9 inch square cake tin. Place them in the oven to heat.

Place the flour in a clean bowl, add the eggs and whisk until smooth. Whisk in the milk and a bit of seasoning until completely smooth.

Remove the hot tins from the oven and pour in equal amounts for the individual muffins are all for the cake tin. Place them back in the hot oven for 20-25 minutes. They should be nicely puffed up and browned. Serve immediately.

These little chappies will also freeze for up to a month. Just take out and re-heat.

Each portion provides 1g protein and 20kcals

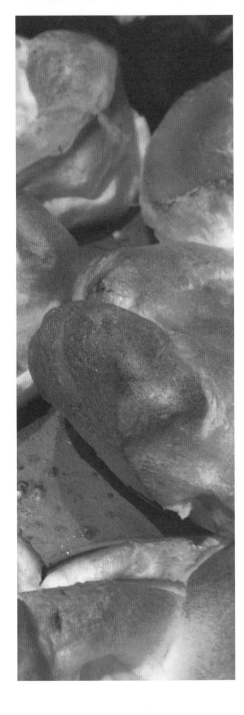

nutrient	thumbs-up score
vitamin B12	👍
sodium	👍
chloride	👍

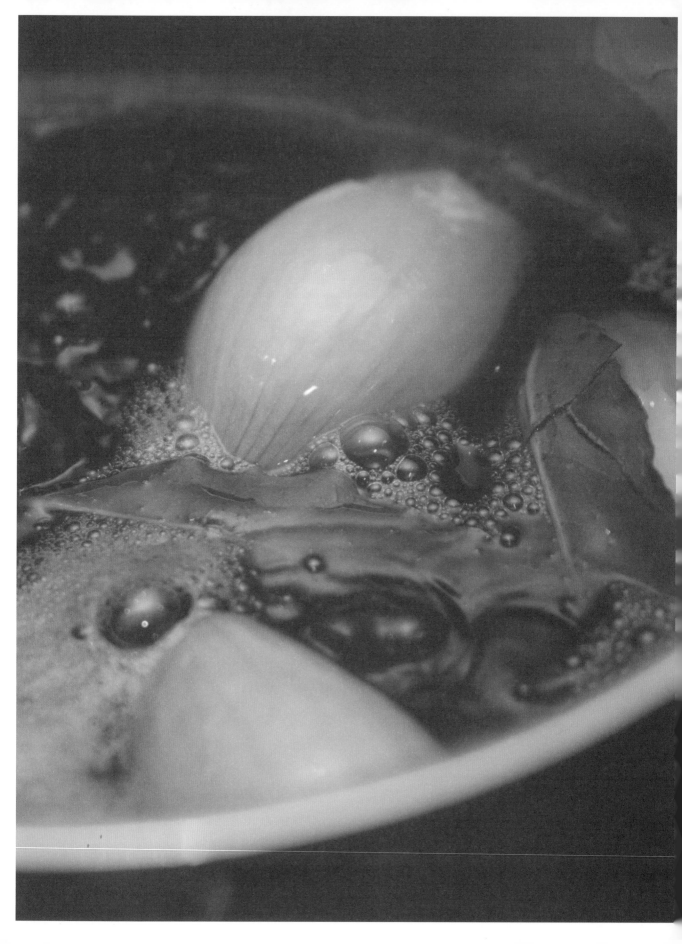

shallot tart

serves 4

This savoury dish is just busting with flavour and is great with game, beef and venison.

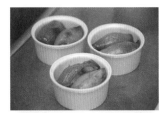

20 small shallots, peeled
2 bay leaves
½ bottle red wine
5 tbsp honey
a few knobs of butter
black pepper
puff pastry, ready made

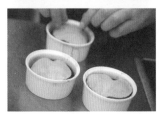

Preheat oven to 170°Cf.

Put the shallots, bay leaves, wine and honey in a saucepan and bring to the boil. Allow to simmer and reduce for 1 hour, then drain the red wine mixture through a fine sieve into a clean saucepan and reduce again until thick. Add butter and black pepper to finish.

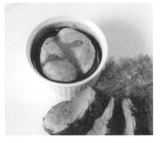

Arrange the cooked shallots into tartlet moulds, 5 to each. Drizzle with the wine mixture then cover with a lid of puff pastry so that the pastry is touching the edges of the sauce. Bake in a bain marie until golden. Remove and drizzle over any remaining sauce to serve.

Each portion provides 6g protein and 380kcals

nutrient   thumbs-up score
The nutritional analysis measures lower than 20% RNI due to small portion size.

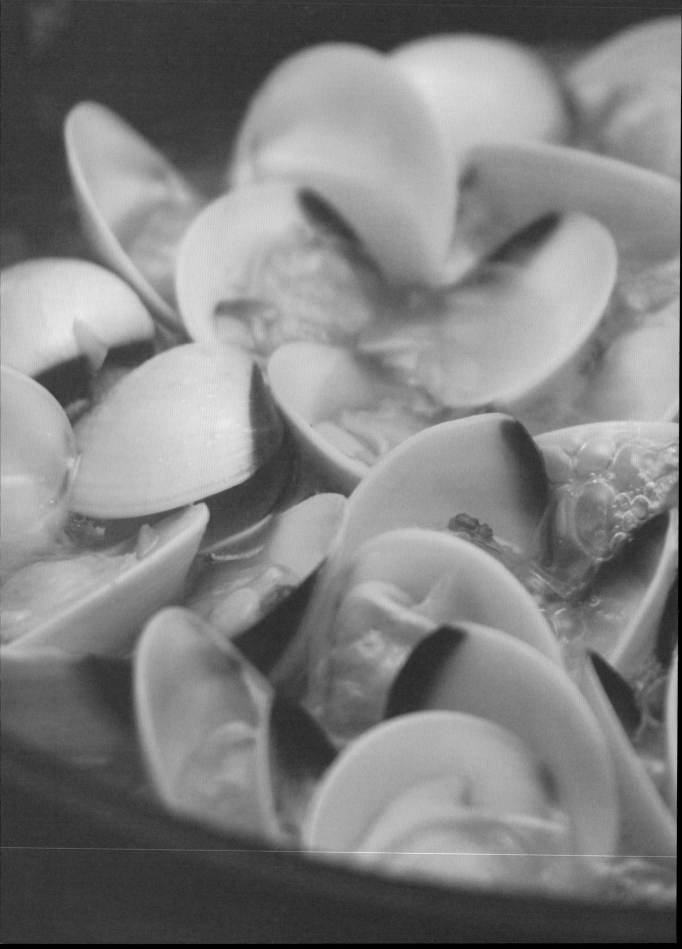

fish & shellfish

fish & shellfish

native canadian wild salmon   179

warm scallop salad   180

baked sea bass with cepes   182

clams in cream & cider   183

seared tuna with green curry sauce   185

trout fillets with tomatoes, ginger & lemongrass   187

grilled sardines with wasabi butter   188

popped oysters   191

fish pie   192

lemon sole & salsa   195

tuna carpaccio   196

escargot   197

pastis prawns on braised fennel   199

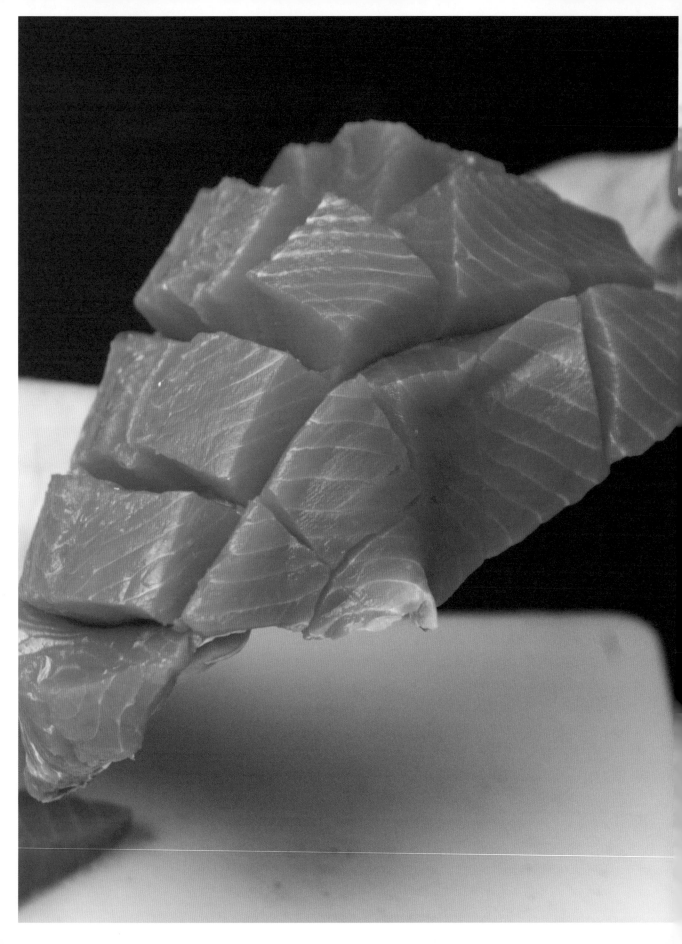

native canadian wild salmon

serves 4

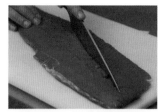

This is a real delight. It originates from the Haida Indians of British Columbia.

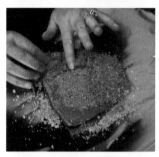

marinade

275g demerara sugar

75g sea salt

25g allspice

25g nutmeg

25g white pepper

3-5 drops liquid smoke* (or a hickory or cedar plank)

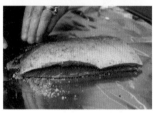

1 salmon, approximately 1.25kg

1 pair needle nose pliers

Fillet the salmon making sure to remove the second ridge of fine bones (thus the pliers). Score the meat into 1½ inch cubes being careful not to break the skin. Mix marinade ingredients then gently rub into the salmon and seal in foil and let marinate for at least 4 hours. If you are using a plank there is no need to add the liquid smoke.

Preheat oven to 180°Cf or a hot bbq.

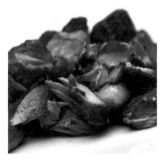

If you are using a plank, remove the fish from the foil and place it on the plank. Put the plank on the bbq grill for 15-20 minutes or until the flesh is just cooked through. If you are baking in an oven, leave the fish in the foil and bake for 20-25 minutes until the fish is cooked through. Timing will vary with the size of the fish.

As an alternative, preheat a bbq to a hot fire and If using a plank, remove from foil and bake for 15-20 minutes.

Serve immediately.

The leftover marinade freezes very well.

Each portion provides 68g protein and 660kcals

* liquid smoke can be bought in most supermarkets in bottle or spray form. I prefer this ingredient to using wood planks

nutrient	thumbs-up score
vitamin B6	>👍👍👍👍
vitamin B12	>👍👍👍👍
vitamin D	>👍👍👍👍
phosphorus	>👍👍👍👍
protein	>👍👍👍👍
selenium	>👍👍👍👍
sodium	>👍👍👍👍
chloride	👍👍👍👍
niacin	👍👍👍👍
thiamin	👍👍
folate	👍
riboflavin	👍
potassium	👍
zinc	👍

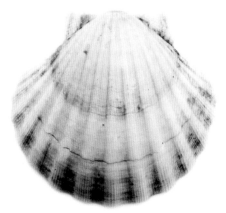

warm scallop salad

serves 4

This is an elegant start for a celebration meal. The scallops are soft and sweet then cherry tomatoes explode with flavour.

16 fresh scallops, hand-dived if available
knob of butter
1 garlic clove, crushed
12 cherry tomatoes on the vine
splash of olive oil
splash of brandy
splash of white wine
mesclun salad*
1 carrot, finely julienned
raspberry vinaigrette†

Wipe the tomatoes with olive oil and place them on a tray in a cool oven long enough to warm through. The skins should slightly split but not colour and don't allow the tomatoes to go soggy.

Arrange the salad on a platter and sprinkle over the carrot and tomatoes.

Melt the butter in a frying pan then sweat the scallops over a medium-low heat until just cooked. Sprinkle over the brandy, flambé then remove the scallops to rest.

Deglaze the pan with the white wine, simmer briefly to reduce then remove from heat and whisk in some raspberry vinaigrette.

Arrange the scallops on the bed of mesclun, drizzle with the dressing and serve immediately.

Each portion provides 24g protein and 360kcals

*see *the basics*, page 281
†see *the basics*, page 282

nutrient	thumbs-up score
vitamin B12	>👍👍👍👍
selenium	👍👍👍
vitamin A total retinol equivalents)	👍👍
phosphorus	👍👍
protein	👍👍
iodine	👍
sodium	👍
chloride	👍
zinc	👍

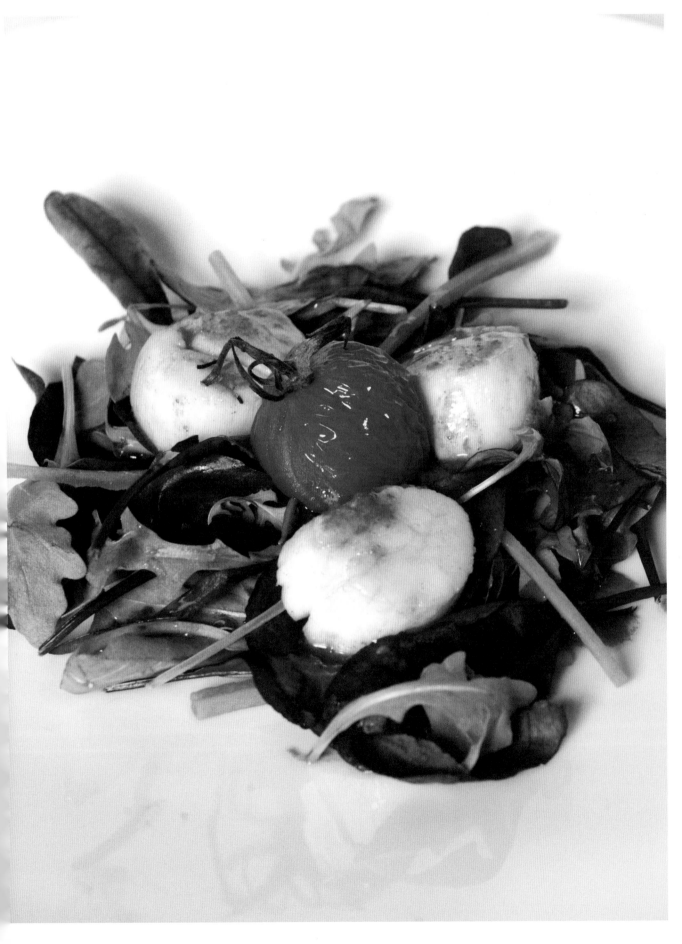

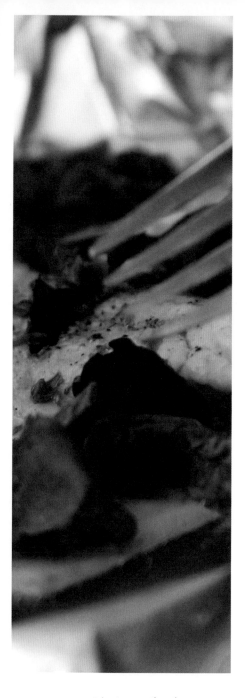

baked sea bass with cepes
serves 4

This is such a lovely way to prepare sea bass. Make sure to seal the foil packets so they are airtight. When you open the pack you get a snoutful of intense wild mushroom aroma…bliss.

4 200g sea bass fillets

50g dried cepes mushrooms

4 bay leaves

small bunch of curly parsley, finely chopped

½ bottle white wine

small splash of white wine vinegar

salt & pepper

knob of butter

Reconstitute the cepes in warm water for at least 2 hours.

In 4 buttered foil packets place the fillets, 6 cepes, 1 bay leaf, a few fingers full of parsley and a dash of salt & pepper. Pour in a few glugs of white wine, a tsp of white wine vinegar and distribute the mushroom infused water amongst the packets.

Preheat the oven to 180°Cf.

Seal the packets tightly, put on a tray and bake for 12-15 minutes. Remove from the oven but keep sealed in packets. Serve in the sealed packets as upon opening you get a poof of rich, steamy heaven.

For an accompanying sauce, prepare a white sauce and add a touch of dijon mustard. This is great served with saffron rice and french beans.

Each portion provides 40g protein and 280kcals

nutrient	thumbs-up score:
vitamin B12	>👍👍👍👍
phosphorus	>👍👍👍👍
copper	👍👍👍👍
protein	👍👍👍
calcium	👍👍
iron	👍👍
vitamin C	👍
niacin	👍
sodium	👍
chloride	👍

clams in cream & cider

serves 4

These are simply divine.

2kg clams, or moules
4 shallots, finely chopped
800ml cider
250ml crème fraiche
knob of butter
small bunch of parsley, finely chopped
salt & pepper

To prepare the clams, rinse them thoroughly in cold water. If using moules, pull away the 'beards' and gently scrape away any barnacles. The shells should be shiny and they should be closed tightly. A good hint is that if they are slightly open they should close when you tap them. Discard any that are dry, float, are wide open or do not smell of fresh sea.

Next, cook half the shallots in butter without colour.

Add the rest of the shallots to 1 pint of boiling water mixed with 600ml cider to steam the clams. This only takes a couple minutes. The shells should open fully and the flesh should be bright in colour.

Strain the clams retaining some of the juice and add a cup of it to the shallots and butter. Add some more cider to the mixture then stir in crème fraiche and let simmer. Season to taste and sprinkle with parsley. Serve with a baguette to mop up the sauce.

Each portion provides 24g protein and 470kcals

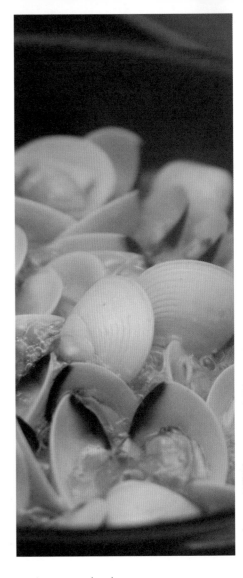

nutrient	thumbs-up score
vitamin B12	>👍👍👍👍
iodine	>👍👍👍👍
iron	👍👍👍👍
selenium	👍👍👍👍
vitamin A total (retinol equivalents)	👍👍
vitamin C	👍👍
riboflavin	👍👍
phosphorus	👍👍
protein	👍👍
sodium	👍👍
chloride	👍👍
vitamin B6	👍
folate	👍
calcium	👍
copper	👍
magnesium	👍
zinc	👍

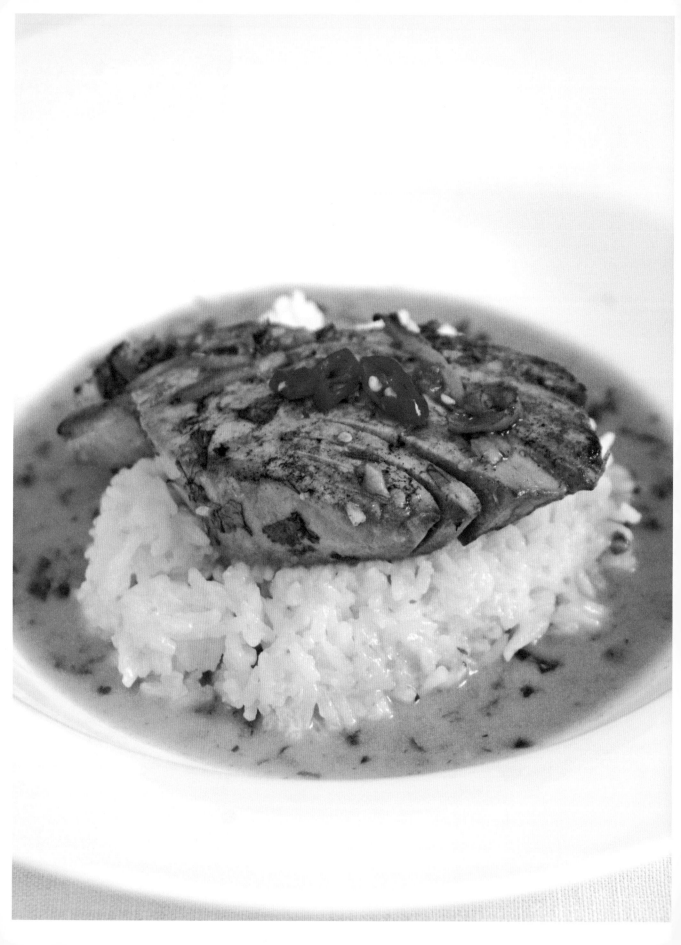

seared tuna with green curry sauce

serves 4

It's a great fish dish when others can be too delicate to taste. Serve it with jasmine coconut rice and sauté of Asian vegetables. It's a wonderful alternative to Sunday roast.

4 175g tuna steaks

green curry sauce

250ml coconut milk

wasabi and ginger pickle for garnish

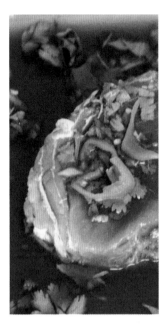

marinade

50ml tamari soy

3 tbsp fish sauce

3 tbsp mirin

a couple drops of sriracha

1 garlic clove, crushed

3cm fresh ginger, peeled and sliced into fine slivers

thai chilli pepper, finely sliced

thai green curry paste

4 tbsp chopped lemon grass

1 tbsp galangal, or ginger as substitute

2 garlic clove, chopped

1 chopped onion

1 large bunch of chopped coriander

juice and zest of 1 lime

2 jalapeno peppers, finely chopped

10 black peppercorns

2 tsp ground coriander

2 tsp ground cumin

2 tsp shrimp paste

1 tsp salt

3 cloves

3 bay leaves

2 tbsp olive oil

nutrient	thumbs-up score:
vitamin B12	>👍👍👍👍
vitamin D	>👍👍👍👍
niacin	>👍👍👍👍
selenium	>👍👍👍👍
vitamin B6	👍👍👍👍
phosphorus	👍👍👍👍
protein	👍👍👍
sodium	👍👍👍
chloride	👍👍
iodine	👍👍
vitamin C	👍
riboflavin	👍
copper	👍
iron	👍
magnesium	👍
potassium	👍

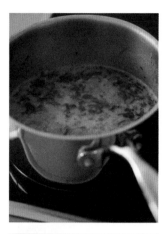

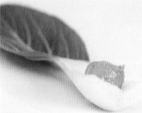

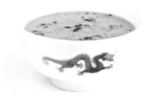

to make the paste

Purée all ingredients into a smooth paste and portion into 4. Keep ¼ portion for use and freeze the rest.

to prepare the dish

Make the curry sauce by heating a quarter of the paste with 250ml coconut milk and water as required. Set aside and warm just before serving.

Prepare the marinade and allow fish to marinate for 30 minutes, covered and put in the fridge. To cook, place steaks on Preheated medium high grill or bbq. Ladle a bit of marinade on the meat. Allow surface to sear, this will only take a minute, Flip the steaks and drizzle with more marinade. Remove when rare to medium rare and rest for several minutes before serving. If you prefer the tuna to be seared and blue, use high heat and flash cook on both sides.

Serve hot drizzled with curry sauce, garnished with wasabi and ginger pickle to finish. Serve with jasmine coconut rice and asian vegetables.

Galangal can be found at most grocery stores. If using fresh, 1 tbsp is equivalent to 2-3 root slices. A 3 inch slice of ginger can be used as a substitute.

Each portion provides 43g protein and 280kcals

trout fillets with tomatoes, ginger & lemongrass

serves 4

These are surprisingly bold flavours for such a delicate fish. The colour is as bold as the flavour.

4 trout filets, skinned

100g italian tomatoes, de-seeded and finely diced

1 large shallot, finely chopped

1 garlic clove, finely chopped

1 small green chilli, finely chopped

1 stick fresh lemongrass, finely chopped

1 tsp fresh ginger, finely chopped

pinch of saffron

24 capers, chopped

1 lime

4 tbsp olive oil

salt & pepper

Preheat oven to 180°C.

Using tweezers, make sure all the fine bones are removed from the fillets. You can find them by gently rubbing your fingers over the flesh. Set in the refrigerator until ready to use.

Add together the tomatoes, shallot, garlic, chilli, lemongrass, ginger, saffron and capers in a bowl. Peel the lime removing all pith and cut into fine wedges removing the membranes as well. Add the lime segments to the mixture.

Season the fillets and place in a lightly oiled baking pan. Top with the tomato mixture then add a cup of water to the bottom of the pan. Bake for 10 minutes. To serve drizzle with the cooking juices and a bit of olive oil.

Each portion provides 24g protein and 150kcals

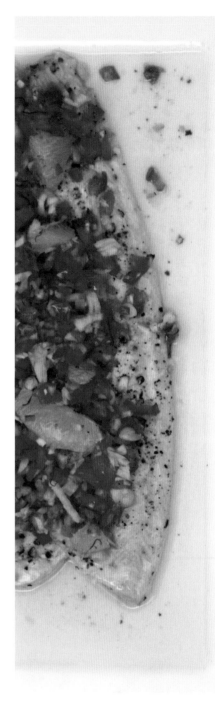

nutrient	thumbs-up score
vitamin B12	>👍👍👍👍
vitamin D	>👍👍👍👍
vitamin B6	👍👍
phosphorus	👍👍
protein	👍👍
vitamin C	👍
niacin	👍
sodium	👍
chloride	👍

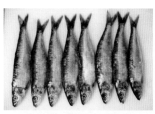

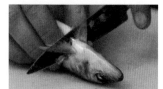

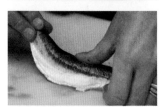

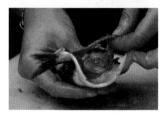

grilled sardines with wasabi butter

serves 4

I love these little bundles of joy. Tiny fish, big flavour.

16 sardines, filleted

sea salt

200g butter

1 tbsp wasabi powder or paste

1 garlic clove, puréed

freshly cracked black pepper

To fillet the sardines, remove the head by prying it gently back and with a small sharp knife slice the length of its underside and remove the innards. Gently pry open the sardine's cavity to butterfly the fish. Run your fingers along the fish's backbone to loosen it from the meat. Starting from the top to the tail, gently lift out the backbone and ribs and remove any stray bones. The tail should pull off with the bones.

Preheat bbq to hot or set oven to grill.

Make the butter by mixing the wasabi, garlic and a few turns of pepper into slightly softened butter. This can be rolled and sealed in cling film and returned to the fridge for storage until ready to use.

Sprinkle salt inside and over the skin of the fish. Place on the bbq or under grill for 1 minute then turn and cook the other side. The skin should go lightly crispy. Serve hot garnished with pats of the wasabi butter.

A super accompaniment for these is the mediterranean fennel salad.

Each portion provides 50g protein and 780kcals

nutrient	thumbs-up score
vitamin B6	>🖐🖐🖐🖐
vitamin B12	>🖐🖐🖐🖐
vitamin D	>🖐🖐🖐🖐
phosphorus	>🖐🖐🖐🖐
selenium	>🖐🖐🖐🖐
protein	🖐🖐🖐🖐
vitamin A total retinol equivalents)	🖐🖐🖐
niacin	🖐🖐🖐
iodine	🖐🖐🖐
sodium	🖐🖐🖐
chloride	🖐🖐🖐
riboflavin	🖐
calcium	🖐
copper	🖐
iron	🖐
magnesium	🖐
potassium	🖐
zinc	🖐

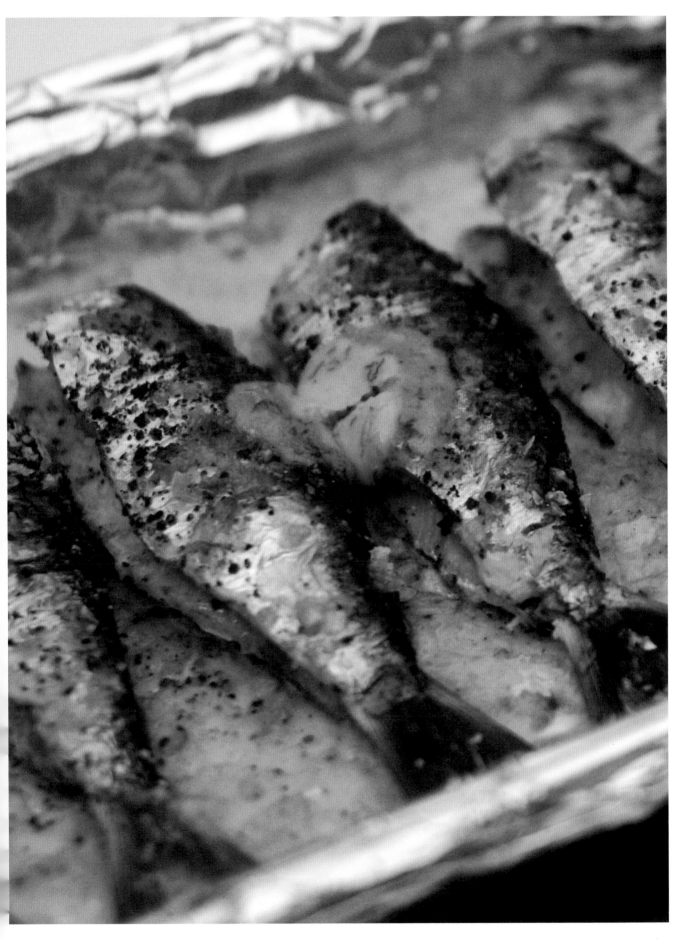

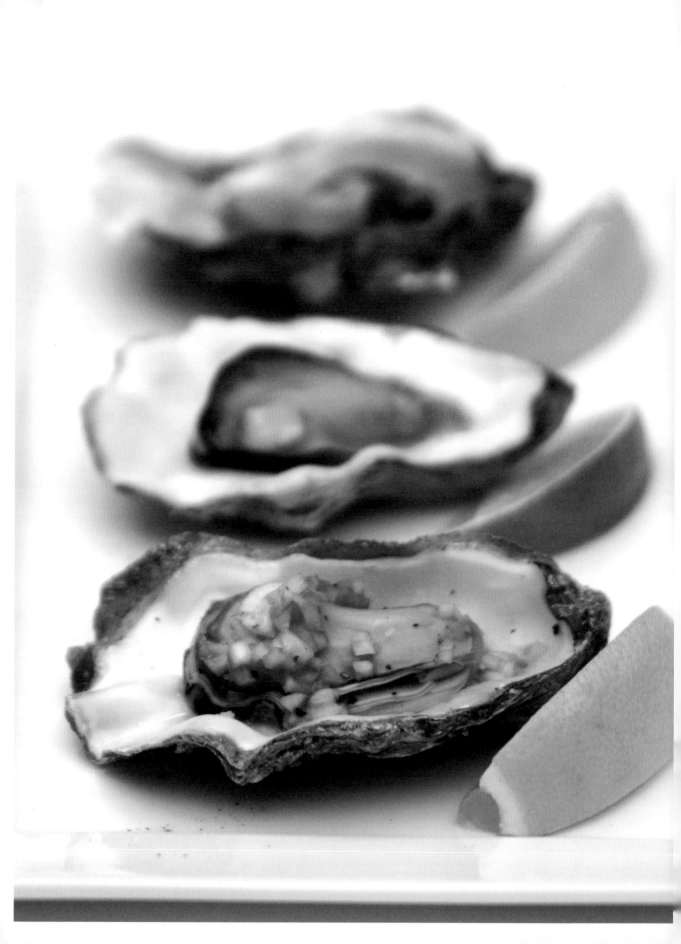

popped oysters

This method takes all the fuss out of preparing oysters, no shucking required. Cooking them in their shell also retains their high nutritional value. Only use oysters that are tightly shut in their shells or close when tapped. Any oysters that stay open should be thrown away.

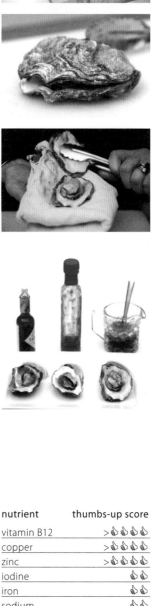

24 fresh oysters
4 lemons, cut into wedges
1 shallot, finely chopped
2-3 pink peppercorns, crushed
3 tbsp white wine
3 tbsp sherry vinegar
tabasco sauce
salt & pepper

Preheat bbq hot or oven to 220°Cf.

To make a traditional mignonette sauce stir together the juice of 1 lemon wedge, shallot, pink peppercorns, white wine and vinegar. Lightly season.

Place the oysters on the bbq grill dish side down. (If in oven place them on a tray.) In about a minute they will 'pop' open. Carefully lift the oysters and using metal tongs pry the upper shell away and discard. The oyster and juices inside will be very hot so protect your hands when working with them. Place on plates with sauces and lemon wedges and serve immediately.

You can control the amount the oysters are cooked so if you like them more on the raw side work very quickly and if you prefer them cooked leave them 30 seconds longer but no more.

Each portion provides 10g protein and 80kcals

nutrient	thumbs-up score
vitamin B12	>👍👍👍👍
copper	>👍👍👍👍
zinc	>👍👍👍👍
iodine	👍👍
iron	👍👍
sodium	👍👍
chloride	👍👍
calcium	👍
phosphorus	👍
selenium	👍

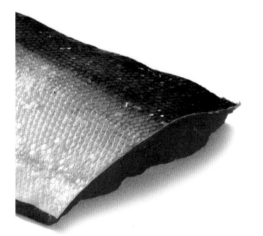

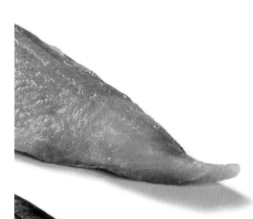

fish pie

serves 4

This is a wonderful dish to pre-prepare for days when things might get a bit hectic or tiring. It's easy to digest.

600ml milk, full fat
1 onion, chopped
2 bay leaves
500g salmon
500g smoked haddock
500g cod or haddock
75g butter
75g plain flour
splash white wine
100ml double cream

7-8 large floury potatoes
1-2 tbsp butter
75ml cream
150g cheddar, grated
nutmeg
salt & pepper

Add milk, onion, bay leaves and a bit of salt & pepper to a large saucepan and warm. Add the fish fillets. Cover and simmer for 2-3 minutes then remove from heat and let stand.

Peel, chop and boil the potatoes then mash adding butter and cream until smooth and fluffy. Add half the cheese and season lightly add a pinch of nutmeg to finish.

Remove the skin from the fillets and tear them into large chunks and place in a casserole. Strain the milk and fish liquid through a sieve into a jug.

Next make a roux*, melting butter in a medium saucepan and stir in the flour. Cook for about a minute on low heat then gradually add the infused milk, wine and cream, stirring over a medium heat for about five minutes. The sauce should be both smooth and thick. Season to taste.

Preheat oven to 200°Cf.

Generously coat the fish with the sauce.

Spoon or pipe the potato over the fish mixture. Start around the outside and ensure that the edges are well sealed with mash then work toward the centre. Fluff the surface with a fork and sprinkle with the remaining cheese.

Place the dish on a baking tray and bake for about 45 minutes or until the top is golden-brown. Allow to rest for 5 minutes before serving.

Each portion provides 95g protein and 1350kcals

*see *the basics*, page 282

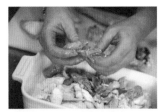

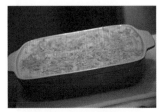

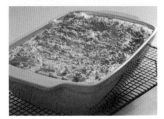

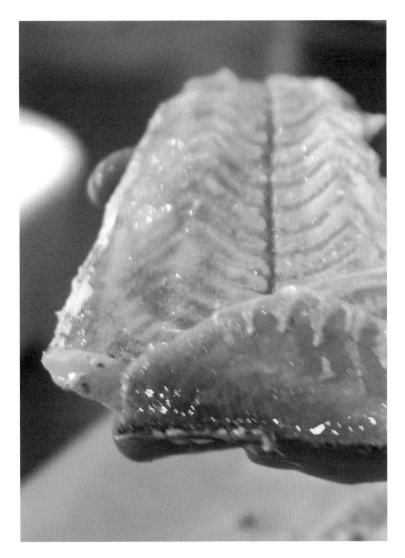

nutrient	thumbs-up score
vitamin B6	>👍👍👍👍
vitamin B12 (by a factor of 10!)	>👍👍👍👍
vitamin A total retinol equivalents)	>👍👍👍👍
vitamin B6	>👍👍👍👍
iodine	>👍👍👍👍
phosphorus	>👍👍👍👍
protein	>👍👍👍👍
selenium	>👍👍👍👍
sodium	>👍👍👍👍
chloride	>👍👍👍👍
calcium	👍👍👍👍
vitamin D	👍👍👍
niacin	👍👍👍
riboflavin	👍👍👍
thiamin	👍👍👍
potassium	👍👍👍
vitamin C	👍👍
folate	👍👍
magnesium	👍👍
zinc	👍👍
copper	👍
fibre (non-starch polysaccaride)	👍
iron	👍

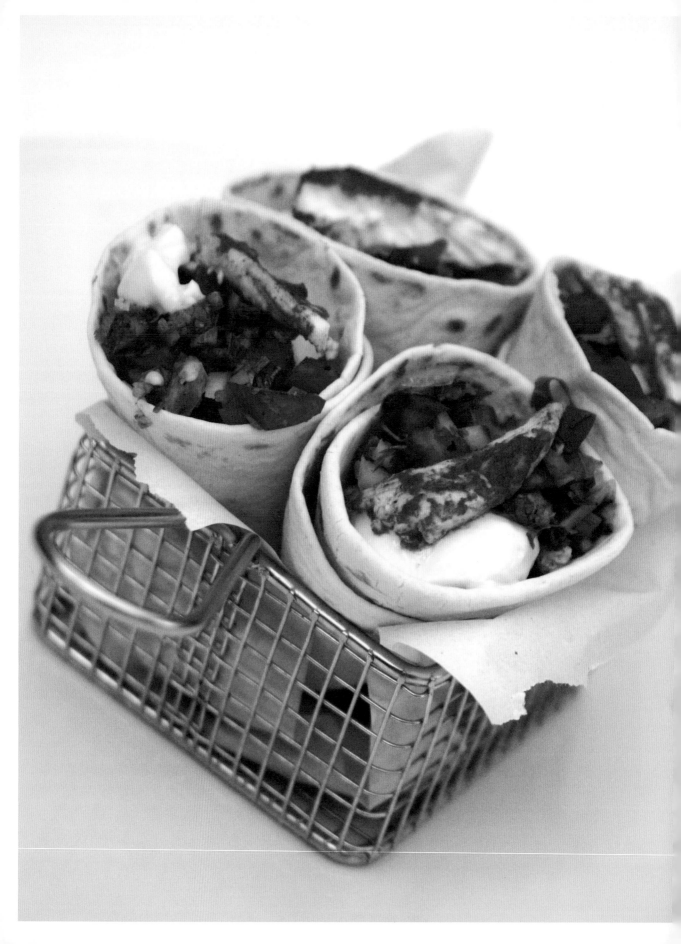

lemon sole fillets & salsa

serves 4

I first came across this dish at a famous cookery school in Cornwall. It's an absolute zinger and makes you think of delicate sole in a completely different way.

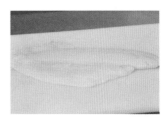

450g lemon sole fillets, skinned
8 flour tortillas
¼ cup mayonnaise*

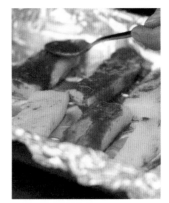

marinade
1 tsp ground cumin
1 tsp hot paprika
2 garlic cloves, puréed
juice of 1 lemon
salt & pepper

salsa
4 tomatoes, seeded & diced
1 small red onion, finely chopped
small bunch of coriander, chopped
1 jalapeno, seeded and finely chopped

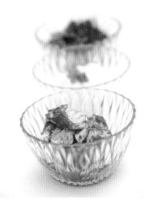

Mix the marinade then coat both sides of the fillets and leave for 20-30 minutes.

Mix the salsa together and season to taste. Gently warm the tortillas in a pan on low heat, about 15 seconds each side and wrap them to keep warm.

Preheat oven to grill (broil) and place the fillets under the grill for 3-4 minutes on one side only. Remove from the heat and break into chunks. Serve with the mayonnaise and salsa in separate bowls with the tortillas and build at leisure!

Each portion provides 29g protein and 530kcals

*see *the basics*, page 281

nutrient	thumbs-up score
vitamin B12	👍👍👍👍
selenium	👍👍👍👍
phosphorus	👍👍👍
sodium	👍👍👍
chloride	👍👍👍
protein	👍👍
vitamin C	👍
niacin	👍
thiamin	👍
calcium	👍
iron	👍

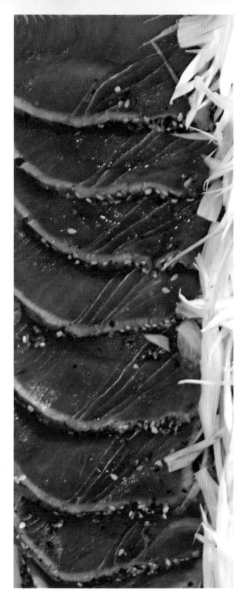

tuna carpaccio
serves 4

Really do try this recipe. It's just so easy and packed with flavour. Don't be afraid that the tuna is raw; it isn't, the citric acid cooks it.

500g piece fresh tuna
juice of 3 lemons or limes
1 tbsp fish sauce
1 tbsp mirin
1 tbsp sesame oil
50g toasted sesame seeds
freshly cracked black pepper
1 shallot, cut into fine slivers
1 fresh chilli pepper, finely chopped
1 small bunch coriander & mint, chopped
tamari soy sauce
wasabi

Combine the lemon/lime juice, fish sauce and mirin in a sealable plastic bag then add the tuna. Place in the fridge and let soak for an hour.

Remove the tuna from the bag and pat dry with a clean towel. The meat should be light brown on the outside and bright, fresh pinky-red on the inside.

Season the sesame seeds with black pepper. Brush the tuna lightly with the sesame oil then roll in the seeds.

Finally, slice the tuna into fine wafers and garnish with the shallot, chilli pepper, mint and coriander. Serve with tamari soy and wasabi for dipping.

Each portion provides 32g protein and 270kcals

nutrient	thumbs-up score:
vitamin B12	>👍👍👍👍
vitamin D	👍👍👍👍
niacin	👍👍👍👍
selenium	👍👍👍👍
vitamin B6	👍👍👍
phosphorus	👍👍👍
vitamin C	👍👍
protein	👍
folate	👍
thiamin	👍
copper	👍
iodine	👍
iron	👍
magnesium	👍
sodium	👍
chloride	👍

escargot

serves 4

This traditional Burgundian dish may seem a little unlikely as a good nutritional source and a healthy dish. It's a perfect starter for beef bourguignon. This is real French comfort food!

24 escargots, cleaned and washed, tinned or frozen

100g butter, softened

3-4 garlic cloves, smashed

2 shallots, finely diced

small bunch of curly parsley, finely chopped

small bunch tarragon, finely chopped

25ml marc du bourgogne, or brandy

pinch of nutmeg

salt & pepper

24 small toasted croutons*, small enough to fit into shells

24 escargot shells

1 small potato, cooked and puréed

sliced baguettes

Preheat the oven to 180°Cf.

Wash the snails in cold water, pat dry and set aside.

Blend the butter, garlic, shallots, parsley, tarragon, marc, nutmeg and seasoning to a smooth and buttery consistency.

Next place a crouton and a small amount of butter mixture into each escargot shell, then add the snail and finish with more butter mixture to fill the remaining cavity.

On ovenproof dishes pipe a dot of potato purée large enough to fix the dressed snail shells, butter side up, 6 to a plate then bake until hot and oozing with melted butter, about 10 minutes. Serve immediately with slices of baguette.

Each portion provides 2g protein and 310kcals

*see *the basics*, page 280

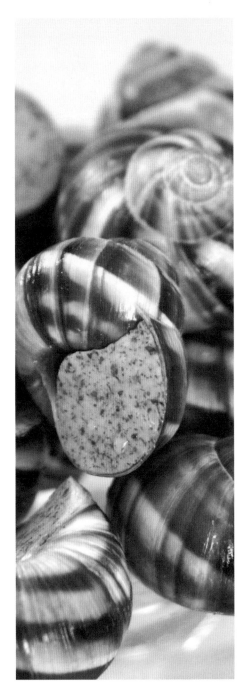

nutrient	thumbs-up score
vitamin A total retinol equivalents)	👍👍
iron	👍👍
sodium	👍👍
chloride	👍
vitamin C	👍
copper	👍
phosphorus	👍
protein	👍
zinc	👍

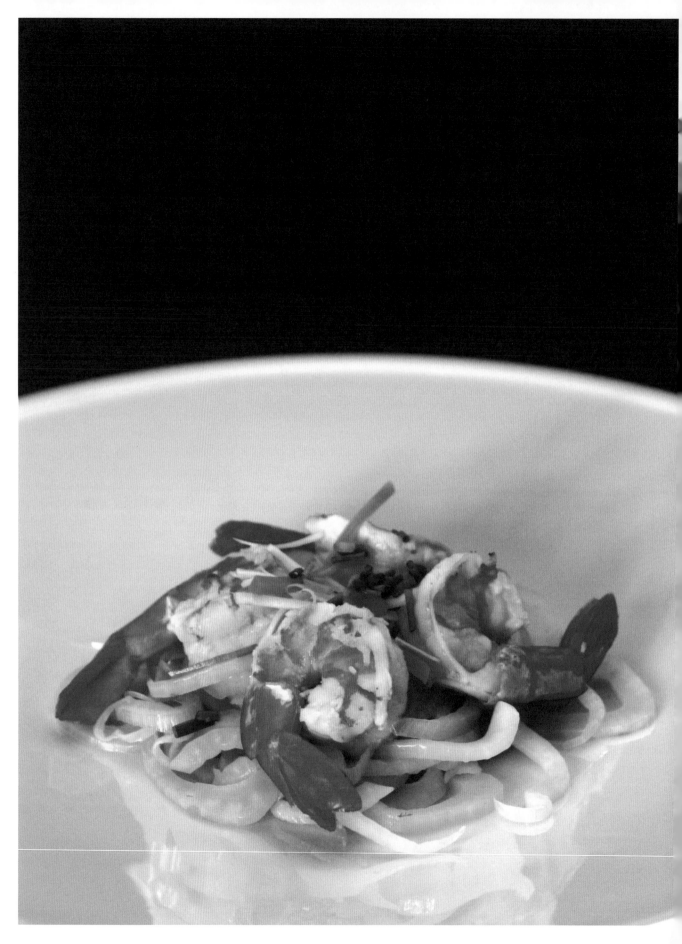

pastis prawns on braised fennel

serves 4 as a starter

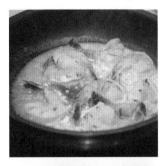

I love this combination of flavours and textures. It's crisp and clean on the palette and beautiful on the plate.

25g butter
1 fennel bulb, finely sliced
50ml white wine
16 large raw prawns, peeled & de-veined
1 garlic clove, crushed
juice of 1 lemon
25ml pastis
chives, finely chopped

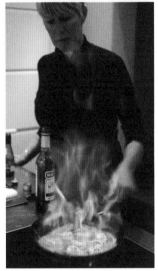

Heat half the butter in a frying pan, add the fennel and white wine and braise until soft. In a separate pan, heat the rest of the butter, garlic and lemon juice until foaming, then add the prawns. Cook until pink then sprinkle over the pastis and flambé. Serve on a bed of braised fennel and sprinkle over the chives to finish.

Each portion provides 23g protein and 185kcals

nutrient	thumbs-up score
vitamin B12	>👍👍👍👍
vitamin A 9total retinol equivalents)	👍👍
phosphorus	👍👍
protein	👍👍
vitamin B6	👍
iodine	👍
iron	👍
selenium	👍
zinc	👍

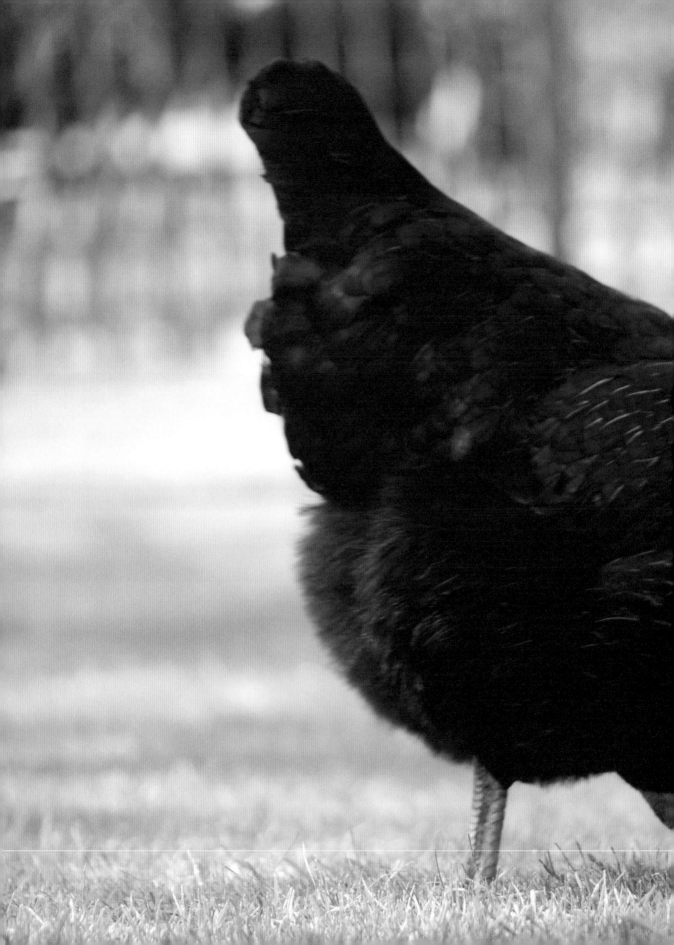

poultry & game

poultry & game

coq au vin	205
chicken, leek & mushroom chasseur	206
breast of duck in tamari marinade	207
provençal lemon chicken	208
christmas turkey smash	211
buffalo wings	212
slow roast pheasant casserole	214
chicken enchiladas	217
chicken garam masala	219
crispy duck pancakes	221
roast quail with celeriac & trompette	222

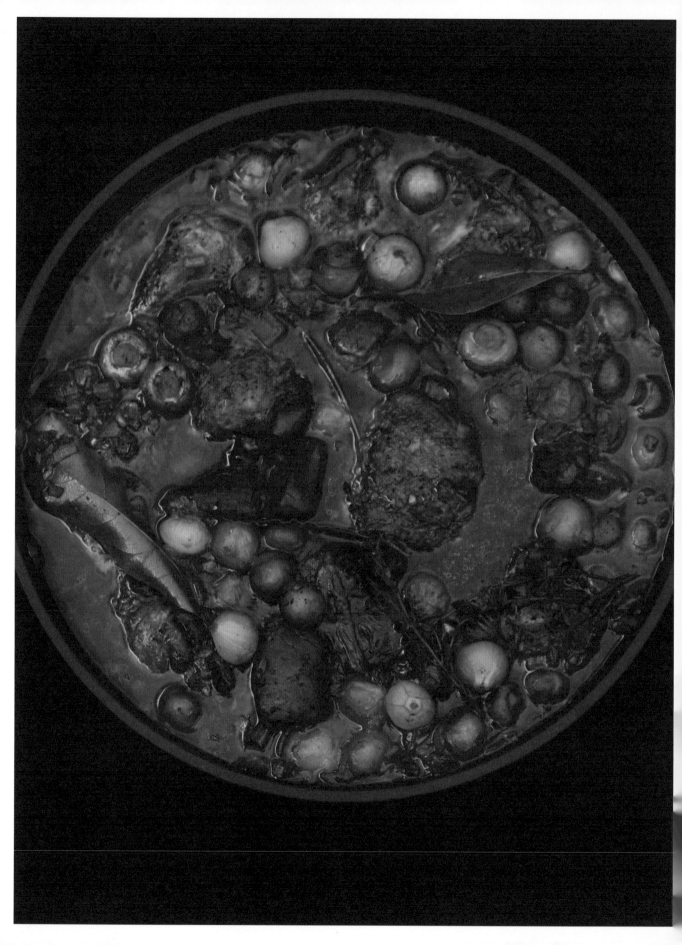

coq au vin
serves 4

This is a great French classic. Preparing it all in one large pan keeps all the goodness in and really saves on the washing up.

1 large corn fed chicken, cut into pieces

150g pancetta

30g butter

2 medium onions, chopped

1 litre hot chicken stock

1 large carrot, chopped

2 stalks celery, chopped

2-3 garlic cloves, chopped

2 tbsp flour

50ml cognac

1 bottle red wine, (burgundy pinot noir preferred)

4-5 sprigs thyme

3 bay leaves

40g butter

12 pearl onions

200g small button mushrooms

Cut the pancetta into small pieces and fry with butter in a deep pan. When golden lift the pancetta into a bowl leaving the fat.

Next season the chicken by rubbing it with salt & pepper and place them in the hot fat and sear them on all sides until golden. The colour of the skin is the key.

Place the chicken with the pancetta. Add the onion, celery, carrot and garlic to the pan. Stir and scrape the residue so that it coats the vegetables. If the mixture gets dry add a bit of stock.

Next return the chicken and pancetta to the pan and stir in flour. Cook for a few minutes then add the cognac and herbs. Finally cover the chicken with wine and stock then add mushrooms and pearl onions. Cover and let simmer for at least one hour or until the chicken is well cooked.

Remove the chicken from pan to rest. Turn up the jus and reduce by half. Add a knob of butter and season to taste.

Each portion provides 120g protein and 940kcals

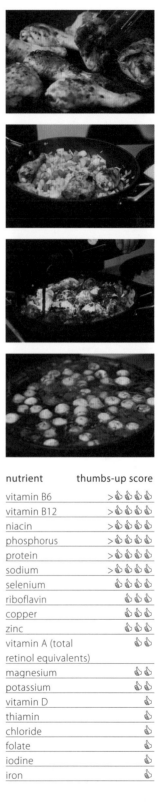

nutrient	thumbs-up score
vitamin B6	>👍👍👍👍
vitamin B12	>👍👍👍👍
niacin	>👍👍👍👍
phosphorus	>👍👍👍👍
protein	>👍👍👍👍
sodium	>👍👍👍👍
selenium	👍👍👍👍
riboflavin	👍👍👍
copper	👍👍👍
zinc	👍👍👍
vitamin A (total retinol equivalents)	👍👍
magnesium	👍👍
potassium	👍👍
vitamin D	👍
thiamin	👍
chloride	👍
folate	👍
iodine	👍
iron	👍

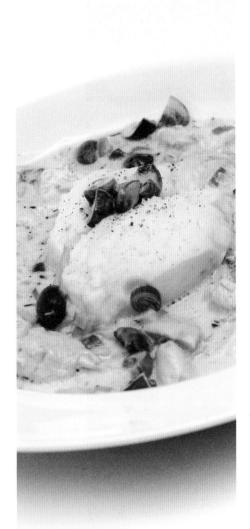

chicken, leek & mushroom chasseur

serves 4

I think I could have this for supper every night.

4 boneless chicken breasts, skinless & cubed
2 garlic cloves, smashed
2 shallots, finely diced
olive oil
splash of brandy
salt & pepper

sauce
200g button mushrooms
1 small leek, white only, thinly sliced
2 shallots, finely diced
120ml white wine
175ml chicken stock
75g crème fraiche
100-150ml single cream, as required
1 tsp dijon mustard
salt & pepper
potato purée to serve
curly parsley, finely chopped for garnish

Heat oil in a large frying pan on medium-high heat and add the garlic and shallots and cook without colour. Add the chicken cubes and cook through until nicely browned. When nearly done, flambé the meat with brandy then remove from heat and set aside to rest.

Next deglaze the pan using a splash of the white wine. Add mushrooms, shallots and leek and cook over medium heat until most of the moisture has evaporated. Now add the remainder of the wine and allow to simmer for a minute then add the chicken stock and allow to reduce by at least half on low heat. Stir in sour cream and mustard and then slowly stir in cream, allowing the sauce to reduce by half. Season to taste.

Add the chicken to the sauce to warm. When ready serve over a potato purée and sprinkle with parsley.

Each portion provides 26g protein and 410kcals

nutrient	thumbs-up score
vitamin B12	>👍👍👍👍
vitamin B6	👍👍👍
sodium	👍👍👍
chloride	👍👍
niacin	👍👍
phosphorus	👍👍
protein	👍👍
vitamin A total retinol equivalents)	👍
riboflavin	👍
copper	👍
potassium	👍
selenium	👍
zinc	👍

breast of duck in tamari marinade

serves 4

This duck breast is super with shallot tart and potato purée. It also works well cold, sliced in a salad like the ichiban slaw.

4 boneless duck breasts, with skin

tamari marinade

250ml red wine
3 tbsp tamari soy sauce
1 tbsp olive oil
1 tsp demerara sugar
juice and zest of 2 limes
dash of sriracha
salt & pepper

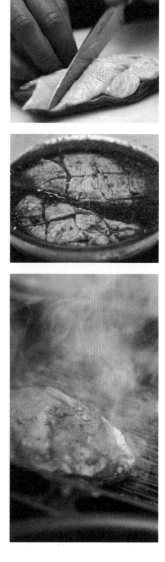

Prepare the duck breasts the day before cooking. Combine the marinade ingredients. Score the skins of the duck breasts without cutting into the meat. Place the duck breasts in a shallow dish or airtight container, pour over the marinade, cover and chill overnight.

To cook, heat a bbq or frying pan until very hot, then place the breasts flesh down and sear. Do not lift or turn the meat until it comes away freely. Just before this point drizzle over a little of the marinade, then turn the breasts and sear the skin side, again drizzling over a little of the marinade.

As the meat browns, drizzle again with marinade. At this point you can turn the breast 45 degrees to create a criss-cross pattern on the skin. Do not allow the skin to burn it should be nicely crisp. Make a final turn to the flesh side, drizzle with marinade and grill for 1 minute or so. Do not over grill as the meat will cook quickly, having marinated for some time.

Remove from heat and allow to rest for five minutes, then slice the meat against the grain. This is great with shallot tart (see page 173).

Each portion provides 24g protein and 170kcals

nutrient	thumbs-up score
vitamin B12	>👍👍👍👍
vitamin B6	👍👍
phosphorus	👍👍
protein	👍👍
sodium	👍👍
chloride	👍👍
niacin	👍
riboflavin	👍
thiamin	👍
copper	👍
iron	👍
selenium	👍
zinc	👍

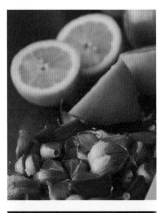

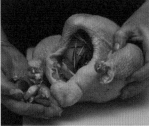

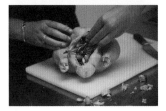

provençal lemon chicken
serves 4

This is an old standby and absolutely divine any time of year. I just love the foolproof simplicity. I serve it with potato dauphinoise. The carcass makes heavenly chicken soup.

1 large corn-fed chicken

2 whole bulbs garlic

8 sprigs rosemary

2 lemons

white wine

flour

1 tsp tomato purée

1 tsp soy sauce

splash of olive oil

salt & pepper

Preheat oven to 200°Cf.

Break up garlic into individual cloves but leave them unpeeled. Halve the lemons. Stuff the chicken with all the garlic, rosemary and lemons then sear it on all sides in a hot pan covered with a thin film of olive oil. Pop the chicken into a roasting pan, cover and place in a hot oven for about 30 minutes then reduce the heat to 160°Cf until well cooked, baste as required or you can bake the bird on its front to allow the juices to run into the breasts in lieu of basting. For the last 4-5 remove the cover and sprinkle with salt. This will ensure a nice golden colour. It's very important to allow the chicken to rest for at least 10 minutes before carving.

Remove stuffing saving the garlic to serve as garnish. Deglaze the roasting tin with white wine adding tomato purée, soy sauce and season to taste. Sift in a small amount of flour and reduce. Strain the sauce through a fine sieve and serve hot.

Each portion provides 95g protein and 1031kcals

nutrient	thumbs-up score
vitamin B6	>👍👍👍👍
vitamin B12	>👍👍👍👍
phosphorus	>👍👍👍👍
protein	>👍👍👍👍
niacin	👍👍👍👍
riboflavin	👍👍👍👍
selenium	👍👍👍👍
zinc	👍👍👍
sodium	👍👍👍
chloride	👍👍
thiamin	👍👍
iron	👍👍
magnesium	👍👍
potassium	👍👍
vitamin A total retinol equivalents)	👍
vitamin D	👍
copper	👍
iodine	👍

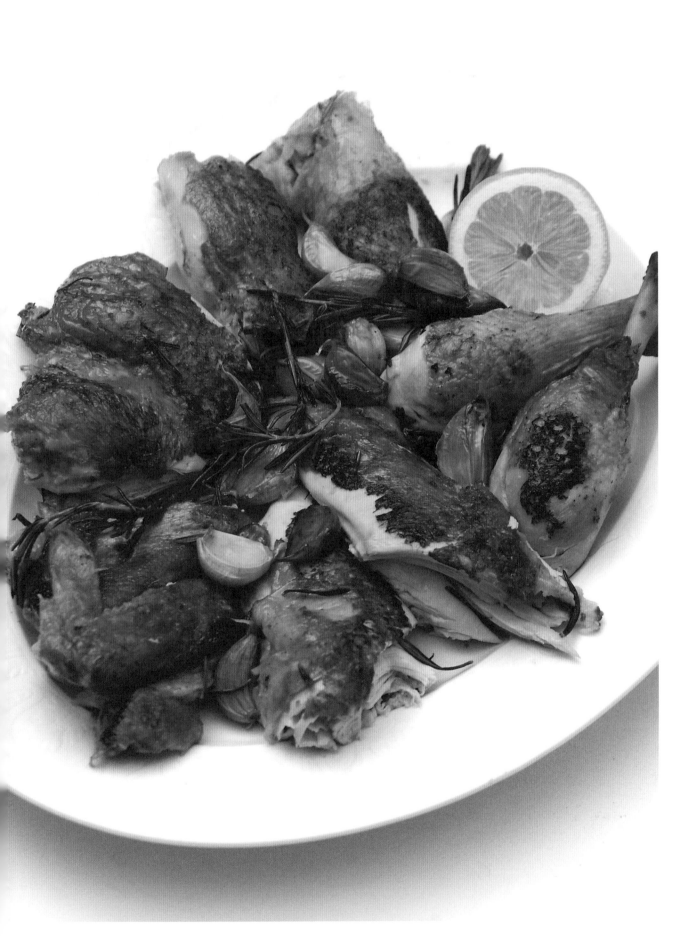

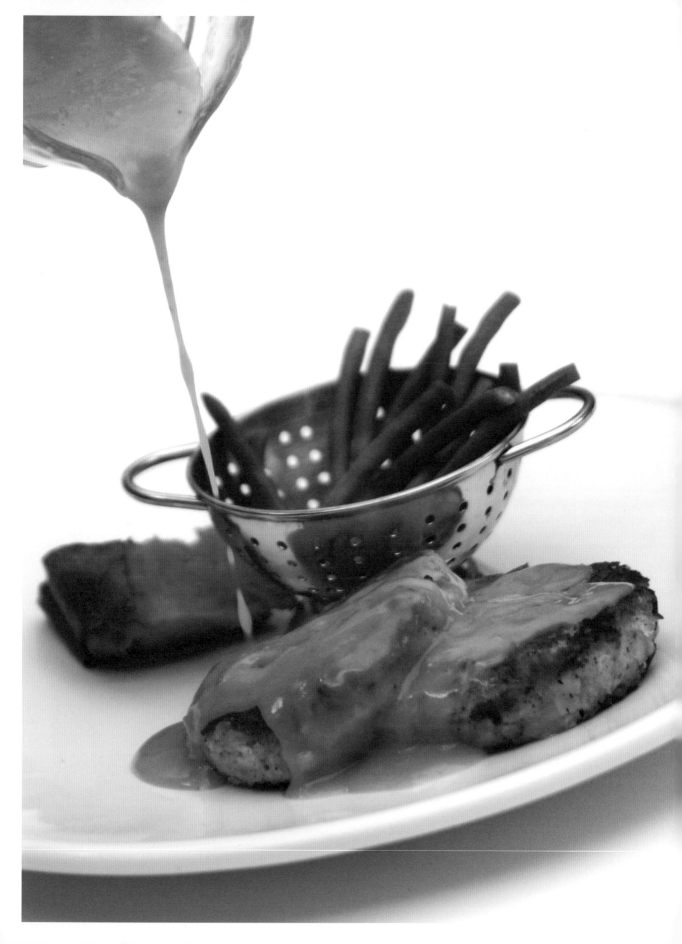

christmas turkey smash

serves as many as you have leftovers for

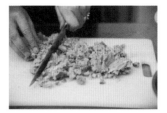

This is the perfect way to finish off the Christmas dinner leftovers. Turkey is an under used and highly nutritious meat. Make this any time of year by roasting a turkey leg and making a stove top dressing.

equal parts of mashed potatoes, stuffing, and chopped turkey
1 egg yolk
1 onion, chopped
2 tbsp butter
a few brussels sprouts or cabbage, cooked and chopped
2 tbsp olive oil
flour for breading the patties
leftover gravy

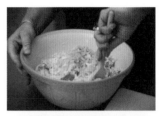

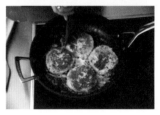

Place the potatoes, stuffing, turkey and egg yolk in a bowl and mix together. Melt butter in a pan and sauté the onion without colour then add the sprouts or cabbage to warm through. Stir the vegetables into the turkey mixture. Form into patties and lightly flour.

Melt a generous knob of butter in a lightly oiled pan and fry the patties on medium heat until crispy golden, turn and crisp the other side. Warm the gravy and drizzle over the patties. Serve hot.

Each portion provides 22g protein and 440kcals

nutrient	thumbs-up score
vitamin B12	👍👍👍
vitamin B6	👍👍
phosphorus	👍👍
protein	👍👍
vitamin A (total retinol equivalents)	👍
vitamin C	👍
folate	👍
niacin	👍
thiamin	👍
sodium	👍
chloride	👍
zinc	👍

buffalo wings
serves 6 (6 pieces per serving)

These are called buffalo wings because they hail from The Anchor Pub, in Buffalo, New York. They are fun little nuggets of happiness for any of life's celebrations.

36 chicken wing pieces, 1 wing makes 2 pieces
1 tbsp sunflower oil
1 tsp salt
225g flour
1½ tbsp white wine vinegar
¼ tsp cayenne pepper
⅛ tsp garlic powder
¼ tsp worcestershire sauce
1 tsp tabasco sauce
¼ tsp salt
6 tbsp louisiana hot sauce
6 tbsp unsalted butter

blue cheese dressing
50g blue cheese
1 garlic clove
1 tsp sea salt
1 tsp mustard powder
juice of ½ lemon
1tbsp balsamic vinegar
2 tbsp olive oil
150ml sour cream
2 tbsp mayonnaise
1 spring onion, finely chopped
salt & pepper
celery sticks for serving

dressing

Purée the garlic and salt together then add the mustard, lemon juice, vinegar and oil. Next blend the sour cream and mayonnaise in a bowl. Thoroughly blend in the oil mixture then whisk in the cheese to desired smoothness. Leave little nuggets of cheese if you want to intensify the flavour. Finally stir in the onion and chill.

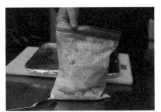

wings

Preheat oven to 220°Cf.

Cut the wings into two pieces, a flat and drum.

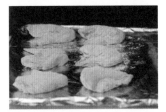

In a bowl toss the wings with the oil, and salt then place in a large sealable bag. Add the flour and shake to coat evenly. Remove wings from the bag, shaking off excess flour, and place on foil-lined baking pans. Try not to crowd them. Bake for about 20 minutes, turn the wings over, and cook another 20 minutes, or until the wings are cooked through and browned.

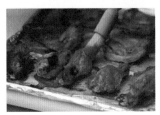

Next mix all the ingredients for the sauce in a pan, and simmer over low heat for about 10 minutes, stirring occasionally.

When the wings are cooked, allow to rest for 10-15 minutes then transfer to a large bowl. Coat the warm wings with sauce and return to the oven for an additional 10 minutes. Serve hot with celery sticks and dressing.

Each portion provides 26g protein and 450kcals

nutrient	thumbs-up score
vitamin B6	👍👍
phosphorus	👍👍
protein	👍👍
sodium	👍👍
chloride	👍👍
vitamin A total retinol equivalents)	👍
niacin	👍
riboflavin	👍
selenium	👍

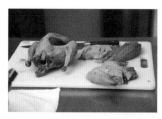

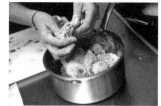

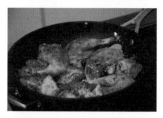

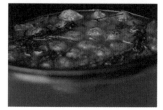

slow roast pheasant casserole
serves 4-6

This rich and luscious winter warmer is good for the sole. Whack everything in the pot and leave it all day. The aroma is half the reward.

1 brace pheasant (2), quartered

20g flour

salt & pepper

splash of olive oil

knob of butter

4 pieces bacon, diced into lardons

2 large shallots, chopped

250ml port

2 tbsp honey

2 whole cloves garlic

2 carrots, chopped

2 parsnips, chopped

2 stalks celery, chopped

20 pearl onions, skinned

3-4 sprigs thyme

500ml chicken stock

Preheat oven to 180°Cf if using a casserole dish or use a slow cooker on medium.

Cut the pheasant into pieces. Check for any stray shot and if there is any really damaged flesh simply cut it away. You can also remove the skin if you prefer a leaner dish. Put the flour, salt & pepper in a sealable bag, add the pheasant and lightly coat.

Melt butter in a lightly oiled pan then brown the pheasant on medium high heat. Remove from the pan then cook the lardons then add the onions and cook without colour. Deglaze the pan with port, add the honey and reduce to half. Return the pheasant and allow to simmer for a further 20 minutes. Season to taste.

Transfer to slow cooker with the carrots, celery, pearl onions and thyme. Cover with stock, seal the lid and slow cook for at least 3 hours. If in a casserole, allow to cook for 1½-2 hours. Serve hot.

Each portion provides 36g protein and 520kcals

nutrient	thumbs-up score
vitamin B12	>👍👍👍👍
vitamin B6	👍👍👍👍
sodium	👍👍👍👍
chloride	👍👍👍
protein	👍👍👍
niacin	👍👍
riboflavin	👍
thiamin	👍
copper	👍
fibre (non-starch polysaccaride)	👍
iron	👍
potassium	👍
zinc	👍

chicken garam masala

This is such a comforting dish any time of year. Prepare it well in advance as a slow cooked dish so the meat is really tenderised.

garam masala spice
50g coriander seeds

50g cumin seeds

20 cardamom pods

10 black cardamom pods

10 blades mace

5 cinnamon sticks, 2 inches

2 tbsp cloves

1 small nutmeg

1 tbsp black peppercorns

4 bay leaves

Place spices on a tray and heat in a cool oven for 3-4 minutes then place in a grinder and whiz to a fine powder.

chicken
250ml chicken stock

1 small onion, finely chopped

2 garlic cloves, smashed

1 tsp ground coriander

5 black peppercorns

1 bay leaf

1 tbsp garam masala

1 tbsp curry powder

1 tbsp tomato purée

juice of 1 lime

4 boneless chicken breasts, skinless

salt & pepper

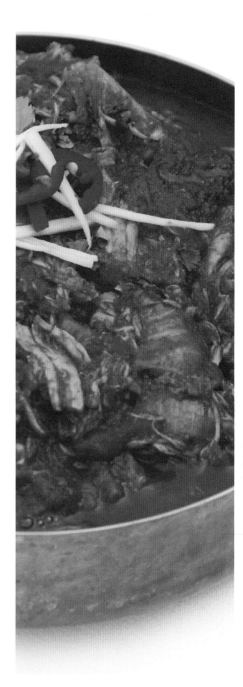

Put the stock, onion, garlic, coriander, peppercorns, bay, garam masala spice, curry powder and tomato purée in a large saucepan and simmer until the onion is soft. Add the chicken filets and lime juice and poach until cooked through. This should take around 20 minutes. Using a wooden spoon gently cut the filets into chunks while they are still in the sauce and keep warm until ready to serve.

Each portion provides 23g protein and 160kcals

nutrient	thumbs-up score
vitamin B6	>👍👍👍👍
vitamin B12	👍👍
phosphorous	👍👍
protein	👍👍
sodium	👍👍
chloride	👍👍
niacin	👍
iron	👍

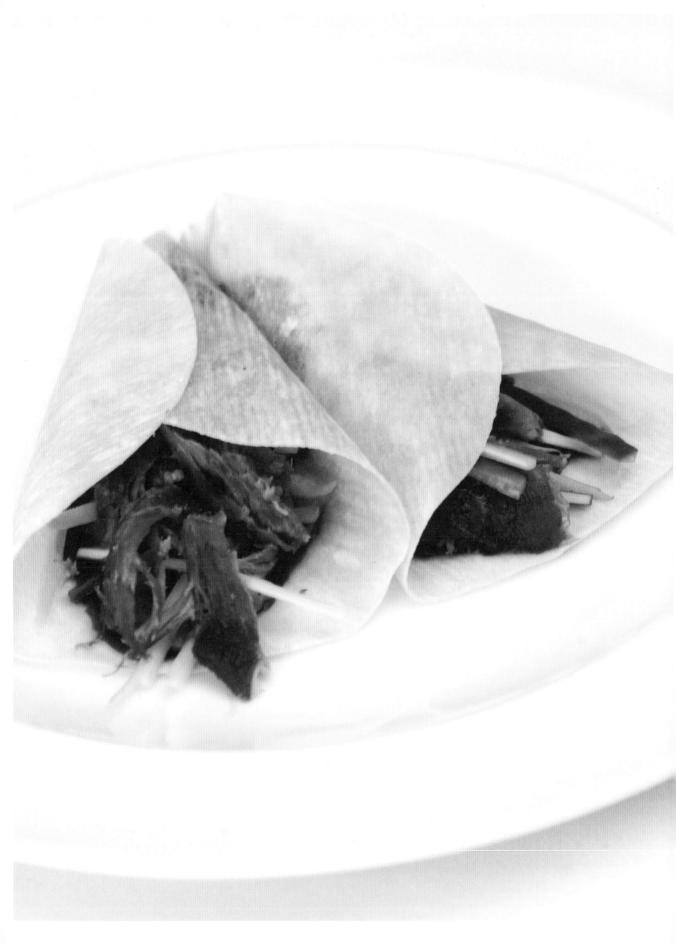

crispy duck pancakes

serves 4

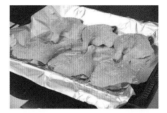

The duck is so easy to prepare. A little goes a long way.

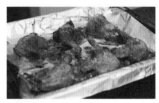

2 duck legs
2-3 handfuls of sea salt
freshly cracked black pepper
4 spring onions, julienned
½ cucumber, seeds removed and julienned
hoisin or plum sauce
chinese pancake wraps

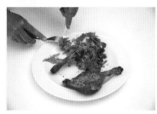

Preheat oven to 220°Cf.

Rub the duck legs generously with salt and place in a deep metal roasting pan. Crack on pepper and place in hot oven for approximately 1 hour. When ready the skin will be dark golden and crackling crisp.

Remove from oven and shred the meat away from the bone with a fork. Serve immediately with onions, cucumber, pancakes and sauce.

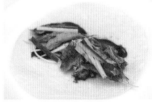

A single duck pancake, assembled on average contains 43g protein and 600kcals*

*In this recipe we have listed nutrients that don't quite make a full 'thumbs-up' in order to demonstrate how much additional nutritional value this snack or light meal contains.

nutrient	thumbs-up score
vitamin B6	>👍👍👍👍
vitamin B12	👍👍👍
phosphorus	👍
protein	👍
sodium	👍
chloride	👍
vitamin A (total retinol equivalents)	3%*
iodine	3%
vitamin C	5%
magnesium	5%
calcium	6%
potassium	6%
thiamin	8%
niacin	9%
copper	10%
iron	11%
selenium	14%
zinc	13%
riboflavin	18%

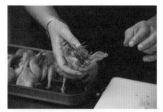

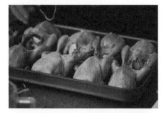

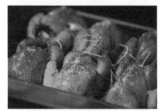

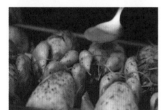

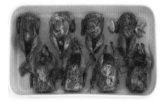

roast quail with celeriac & trompette

serves 4

This dish serves the quail whole, which can be a bit fiddly to eat but delicious. They are small and fast to prepare so there is less preparation time. It's a lovely Sunday lunch.

4 quail
8 large garlic cloves, whole and unpeeled
1 lemon
bunch of rosemary
2 bay leaves
50g clarified butter
250ml white wine
salt & pepper

1 celeriac, diced into small cubes
large knob of butter
1-2 tbsp single cream
small bunch of chives, finely chopped
handful of trompette mushrooms, or other fine wild mushrooms
splash of olive oil
splash of red wine vinaigrette*

Preheat oven to 180°Cf.

Slice the lemon into small pieces (about ½ inch). Stuff the quail with 2 garlic cloves, 2 pieces of lemon and a couple sprigs of rosemary and place in a roasting pan with a few more lemon pieces, bay leaves and lightly season. Next drizzle the birds with the clarified butter, cover with tin foil and roast for about 10 minutes.

Lower the oven temperature to 160 degrees C and remove the cover from the birds. Pour the wine over the birds and return to the oven for another 20 minutes. Baste about half way through. Remove the birds when fully cooked and golden. Allow to rest for 5 minutes before serving.

For the celeriac, melt butter in a pan then add diced celeriac and

nutrient	thumbs-up score
vitamin B12	>👍👍👍👍
vitamin B6	👍👍👍
phosphorus	👍👍
protein	👍👍
vitamin A (total retinol equivalents)	👍
vitamin C	👍
niacin	👍
riboflavin	👍
copper	👍
iron	👍
selenium	👍

sauté until soft. Add the cream and chives, warm through and set aside.

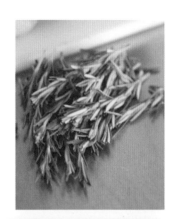

For the mushrooms, lightly coat a pan with oil on medium high heat then add the mushrooms. Sauté long enough for the moisture to evaporate. This will intensify the flavour of the mushrooms. To finish, add a splash of red wine vinaigrette.

Each portion provides 29g protein and 400kcals

*see *the basics*, page 282

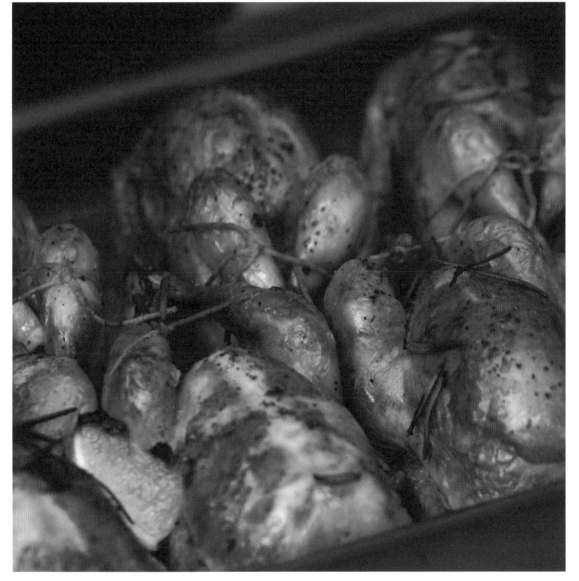

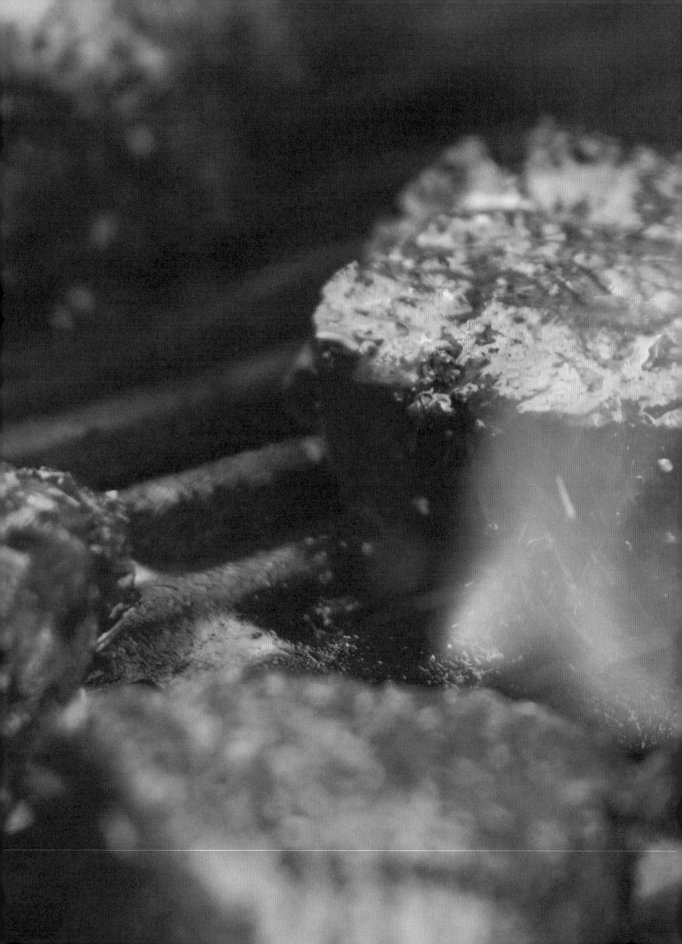

beef, lamb, pork & venison

beef, lamb, pork & venison

beef bourguignon   229

medallions of aberdeen angus & mushroom duxelle   230

filet of venison & chocolate jus   231

warm beef salad & raspberries   232

simon's pie   235

pork tenderloin piri piri   236

escallop of veal & pink peppercorn sauce   237

cabbage rolls   239

lamb keema kaleji   240

welsh cawl   243

beef teriyaki brochettes   244

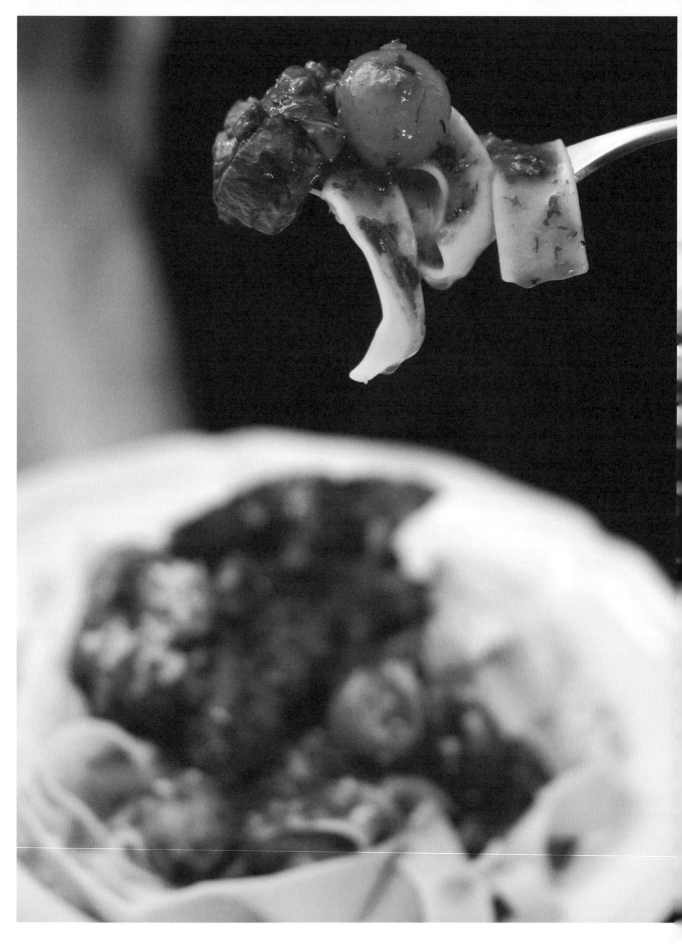

beef bourguignon

serves 6-8

This is possibly one of the best meals ever invented. As a slow cooked dish it really takes very little effort to produce a magnificent meal.

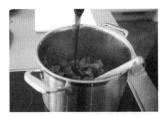

olive oil

3 garlic cloves, crushed

dash of sriracha

1 bottle red burgundy

350g steak, cubed

15-20 pearl onions, peeled

15-20 small button mushrooms

herbs de provençe

2 tbsp dijon mustard

salt & pepper

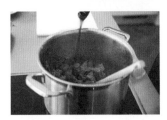

egg tagliatelle

parmesan cheese, finely grated

sliced baguette to serve and mop up the gravy

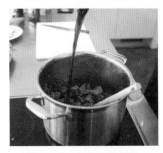

In a deep saucepan, warm the garlic and sriracha in a little olive oil. Splash in a little wine, add the beef then turn up the heat and sear all over. Reduce heat then add onions, mushrooms and the bottle of wine. Simmer for at least an hour, adding salt, pepper and herbs to taste.

Then add the mustard, a few extra herbs and the rest of the wine and simmer for another hour. Stir from time to time and season to taste.

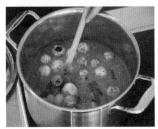

Prepare the noodles al dente* and rinse well. This is a communal dish so serve the pasta and beef in separate bowls with bread and cheese on the side and let everyone dive in.

Each portion provides 21g protein and 245kcals

*see *the basics*, page 280

nutrient	thumbs-up score
vitamin B12	👍👍👍
vitamin B6	👍👍
copper	👍👍
phosphorus	👍👍
iodine	👍
iron	👍
protein	👍
selenium	👍
sodium	👍
chloride	👍
zinc	👍

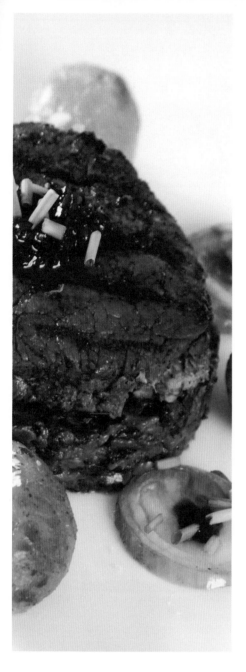

medallions of aberdeen angus & mushroom duxelle

serves 4

This is straightforward, rich and delicious. There is no need to mess with a fine piece of fillet and the duxelle adds bags of flavour and nutrition.

750g beef tenderloin, 4 medallions

1½ tsp sea salt

1½ tbsp freshly cracked black pepper

splash of red wine

marinade

3 tbsp olive oil

2 tbsp lemon juice

1½ tbsp beef stock

1½ tbsp soy sauce

1 tbsp white wine vinegar

¾ tsp sugar

1 garlic clove, puréed

Prepare marinade. Cut tenderloin into 3cm medallions. Crack pepper onto a plate then pat the medallions into the pepper leaving a light coat. Sprinkle with salt then place in marinade for 1 hour.

Sear in a hot pan to desired finish (rare). Allow to rest for several minutes before serving.

Deglaze the pan with red wine and reduce. Serve on bed of mushroom duxelle (see page 164).

Each portion provides 40g protein and 270kcals

nutrient	thumbs-up score
vitamin B12	>👍👍👍👍
vitamin B6	👍👍👍
phosphorus	👍👍👍
protein	👍👍👍
sodium	👍👍👍
chloride	👍👍👍
zinc	👍👍
niacin	👍
riboflavin	👍
thiamin	👍
iron	👍
potassium	👍

fillet of venison & chocolate jus

serves 4

Venison is leaner than beef and has a stronger and richer flavour. Also, it takes about 30 minutes for alcohol to fully dissipate so take your time preparing the sauce and allow the meat to fully rest before serving.

marinade

50ml olive oil

50ml red wine

juice of 2 limes

1 garlic clove, puréed

1 shallot, finely chopped

dash of sriracha

1 bay leaf

handful of herbs de provençe

salt & pepper

1 venison tenderloin

25ml cognac

250ml red wine

50g 70% chocolate, grated finely

freshly cracked black pepper

knob of butter

Marinate the venison for at least 1-2 hours.

Cut tenderloin into 1½ inch medallions. Coat both sides with cracked black pepper. Sear tenderloin on both sides on a very hot flying pan. Continue to grill and douse with marinade while cooking. Use all the marinade in this process as it makes the base for the jus. To finish, flambé the meat with cognac. Remove from heat and allow to rest.

For the chocolate jus, deglaze the skillet by adding red wine and reduce by half. Pass this mixture through a fine sieve into a pan and continue to reduce adding wine as needed. Add chocolate stirring constantly. And finally add knob of butter to finish.

Each portion provides 46g protein and 490kcals

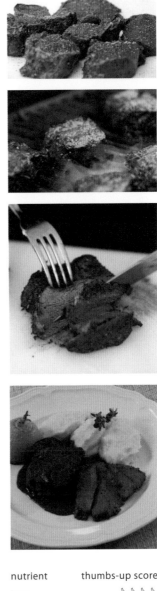

nutrient	thumbs-up score
iron	👍👍👍👍
phosphorous	👍👍👍👍
protein	👍👍👍👍
copper	👍👍
sodium	👍👍
zinc	👍👍
riboflavin	👍
chloride	👍
magnesium	👍
potassium	👍
selenium	👍

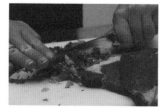

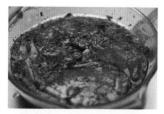

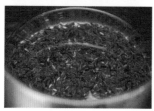

warm beef salad & raspberries

serves 4 as a main

This is a lovely way to serve beef. Perfect for chemo days, as the beef is prepared well in advance and can be dished up without fuss. The marinade adds a lot of flavour.

500g flank steak

camargue red rice, use wild rice if not available

chicken stock

lamb's lettuce

raspberries

walnut halves

marinade

150ml olive oil

300ml red wine

herbs de provençe

3-4 cloves of garlic, crushed

juice of 4 limes

small bunch of fresh coriander, chopped

dash of sriracha

salt & pepper

Combine the marinade ingredients in a shallow dish. Add the steak and marinate for at least 2 hours.

Remove the meat from the marinade, then grill or bbq to medium rare. Allow to rest for 15 minutes before slicing thinly against the grain. The meat should have a criss-cross pattern. This will prevent the meat from being tough. Seal in an airtight container and refrigerate overnight.

Cook the rice in stock instead of water. To serve, spread the rice on a large platter, surround with lamb's lettuce and sprinkle with the raspberries and walnut halves. Fan the slices of beef over the rice. Drizzle with raspberry vinaigrette.*

Each portion provides 35g protein and 580kcals

*see *the basics*, page 282

nutrient	thumbs-up score
vitamin B12	>👍👍👍👍
vitamin B6	👍👍👍
protein	👍👍👍
zinc	👍👍👍
phosphorus	👍👍
sodium	👍👍
chloride	👍👍
vitamin C	👍
iron	👍

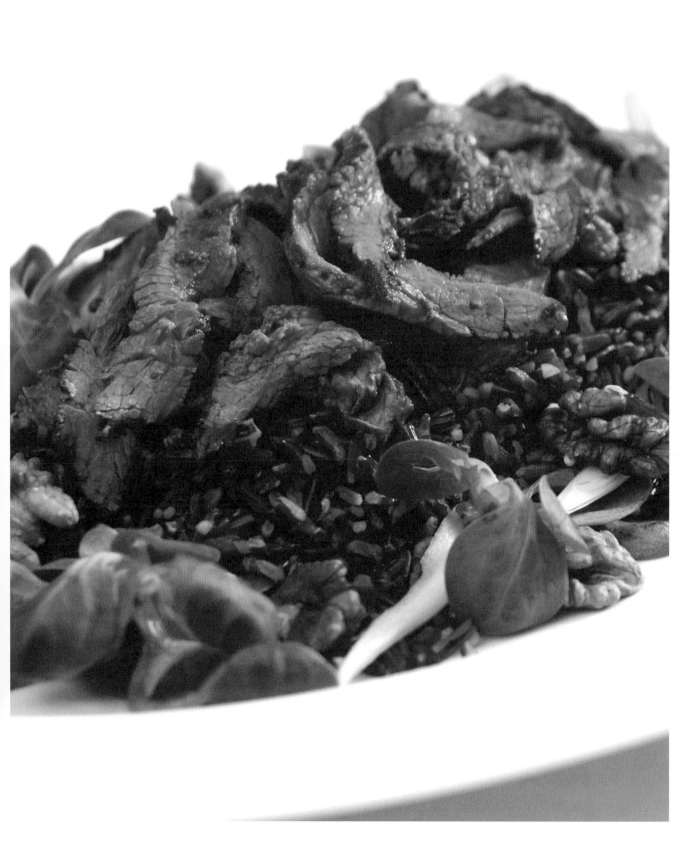

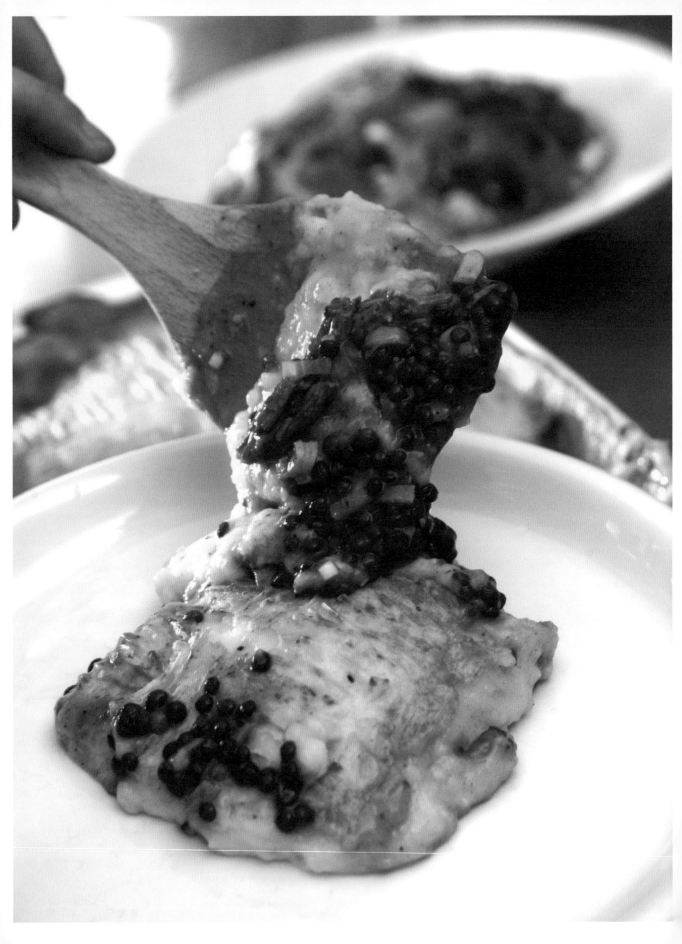

simon's pie

serves 4-6

This is a really nutritious take on shepherd's pie. I made up this dish when Simon was in chemotherapy. It's perfect to come home to.

4 lamb shanks
2 tsp olive oil
1 bottle of red wine
6 garlic cloves
2 onions, chopped
a generous handful of mixed herbs
500ml lamb stock
dash of sriracha
salt & pepper
3 bay leaves

1.25 kg potatoes
2 to 3 tsp white plain flour
100ml water, approximately
200g shallots, finely chopped
800g pre-cooked puy lentils, 2 tins
nutmeg

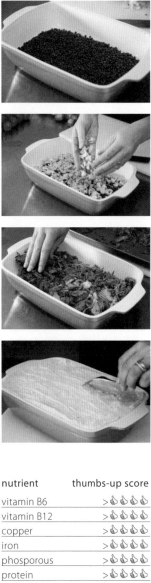

Slow cook the lamb and ingredients on medium for 6-8 hours. The meat should fall off the bone. When ready strain the jus through a fine sieve. Pull from the bones ensuring there is no fat. Next boil and mash potatoes and season with salt, pepper and nutmeg.

To make the gravy, bring the jus to hard boil then reduce heat to simmer. Using flour and water, make a smooth paste and whisk into the jus avoiding lumps. Bring back to the boil. Season to taste.

Preheat oven to 200°Cf.

Finally, layer the lentils, shallots and lamb in a casserole. Add sufficient gravy to completely cover the meat then cover with a generous layer of potatoes adding seasoning and a dash of nutmeg. Seal to the edges to prevent the sauce from boiling over. Rough up the surface using a fork. Bake until golden brown on top. Remove from heat and leave to rest for 10 minutes before serving.

Each portion provides 77g protein and 1080kcals

nutrient	thumbs-up score
vitamin B6	>🥄🥄🥄🥄
vitamin B12	>🥄🥄🥄🥄
copper	>🥄🥄🥄🥄
iron	>🥄🥄🥄🥄
phosporous	>🥄🥄🥄🥄
protein	>🥄🥄🥄🥄
selenium	>🥄🥄🥄🥄
zinc	>🥄🥄🥄🥄
thiamin	🥄🥄🥄🥄
fibre (as non-starch polysaccharide)	🥄🥄🥄🥄
vitamin C	🥄🥄🥄
folate	🥄🥄🥄
niacin	🥄🥄🥄
magnesium	🥄🥄🥄
riboflavin	🥄🥄
sodium	🥄🥄
chloride	🥄🥄
calcium	🥄

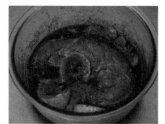

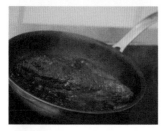

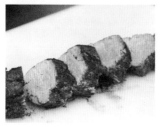

pork tenderloin piri piri
serves 4

This is just a wonderful way to serve pork. The marinade gives the meat bags of flavour without taking away the delicacy of the tenderloin. It's also perfect on the bbq.

1 pork tenderloin

marinade

3 chilli peppers, finely chopped, leave the seeds in for heat

juice of 2 lemons

3 garlic cloves, minced

small bunch of parsley, chopped

3-4 tbsp paprika

4 tbsp olive oil

300ml white wine

salt & pepper

Mix all ingredients of marinade together and place tenderloin in a dish, cover, place in refrigerator and allow to soak for at least 1-2 hours. No need to rush.

On a hot bbq sear the tenderloin on all sides allowing to colour without burning. You will know when to turn, as the meat will lift from the grill. If it doesn't, it's not ready.

Lower the heat and continue to grill basting with marinade regularly. Once seared marinate generously then roast in a preheated oven at 180°Cf for approximately 30 minutes. Cook to the rare side of medium then allow to rest for at least 5 minutes. When sliced it should be cooked through but still just pink inside.

Each portion provides 24g protein and 240kcals

nutrient	thumbs-up score:
vitamin A (total retinol equivalents)	>👍👍👍👍
thiamin	👍👍👍👍
vitamin B6	👍👍
vitamin B12	👍👍
phosphorus	👍👍
protein	👍👍
vitamin C	👍
niacin	👍
riboflavin	👍
iron	👍
magnesium	👍
potassium	👍
selenium	👍
sodium	👍
chloride	👍
zinc	👍

escallop of veal & pink peppercorn sauce

serves 4

This is the meal you want to prepare when the boss and his wife come to dinner. A real classic. Serve with roasted new potatoes and stuffed globe courgette.

8 75g medallions of veal
600ml whipping cream
50ml brandy
25 white wine
2 tsp pink peppercorns
salt & pepper
splash of olive oil
knob of butter
drop of sriracha
1 large shallot, finely chopped

Place a small amount of oil and knob of butter in a hot frying pan. Lightly flour veal medallions and place in the skillet when butter is bubbling. Quickly fry on both sides leaving the veal medium rare. Remove the veal and let rest.

Add the shallot to the pan and fry for 2 minutes then add the wine and brandy and flambé. Crush the pink peppercorns with the back of a knife and add these and the cream to the deglazed pan. Reduce until the liquid becomes thicker then add a drop of sriracha and salt & pepper. Drop in a knob of butter then place the veal and juices into the sauce and cook on medium heat for 2 minutes. Serve immediately.

Each portion provides 37g protein and 780kcals

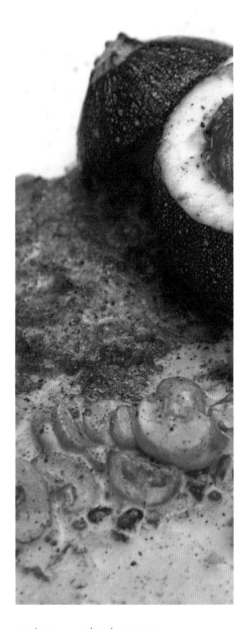

nutrient	thumbs-up score
vitamin B12	>👍👍👍👍
vitamin B6	>👍👍👍👍
vitamin B12	>👍👍👍👍
vitamin A (total retinol equivalents)	👍👍👍👍
phosphorus	👍👍👍👍
protein	👍👍👍
niacin	👍👍
riboflavin	👍👍
zinc	👍👍
vitamin D	👍
potassium	👍
sodium	👍
chloride	👍

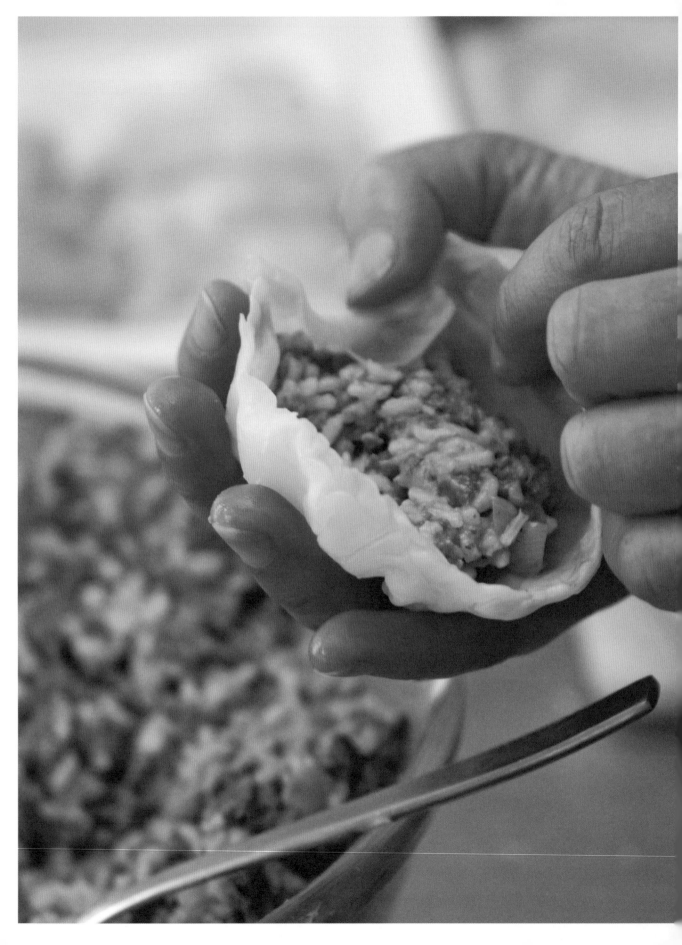

cabbage rolls (golabki)

serves 4

This is a wonderful traditional Polish meal. Don't be put off by school meal memories of boiled cabbage. It's absolutely packed with flavour.

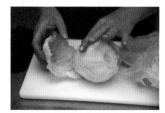

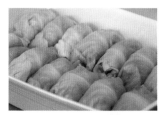

1 head white cabbage

225g long grain white rice, uncooked

3-4 garlic cloves, crushed

1 dash sriracha

1 large onion, finely chopped

450g beef mince

225g pork mince

2 tbsp mixed herbs

1 tbsp paprika

3 tbsp worcestershire sauce

2 eggs, beaten

salt & pepper

1 litre passata

400g chopped tomatoes

salt & pepper

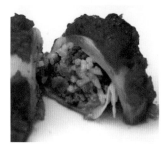

Remove the core from the cabbage and place in simmering water. As the cabbage softens remove the leaves being careful not to break them. This will take about 40 minutes. The innermost leaves will be too small to use and can be finely chopped and added to the meat mixture. The cabbage is hot so take precautions.

To make the filling, cook the rice and warm the garlic and chilli paste in an oiled skillet. Add onions and cook without colour. Sauté the mince with the garlic and onions and add herbs, paprika and worcestershire sauce. Season to taste. When fully cooked, add the meat and rice together then stir in the eggs. Check the seasoning.

For the sauce add passata, tomatoes, garlic and seasoning together in a pan. Allow to simmer for about 20 minutes.

Preheat oven to 160°Cf.

To make the rolls, place a scoop of the meat into the centre of a cabbage leaf and roll, then place opening down into a casserole. Ladle the sauce over the rolls and bake in a low oven for an hour.

Each portion provides 46g protein and 840kcals

nutrient	thumbs-up score
vitamin A (total retinol equivalents)	>👍👍👍👍
vitamin B6	>👍👍👍👍
vitamin B12	>👍👍👍👍
phosphorous	👍👍👍👍
protein	👍👍👍👍
sodium	👍👍👍👍
chloride	👍👍👍👍
vitamin C	👍👍👍
niacin	👍👍👍
thiamin	👍👍👍
iron	👍👍👍
zinc	👍👍👍
potassium	👍👍
vitamin D	👍
riboflavin	👍
calcium	👍
copper	👍
fibre (as non-starch polysaccharide)	👍
folate	👍
iodine	👍
magnesium	👍
selenium	👍

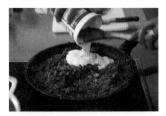

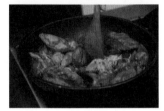

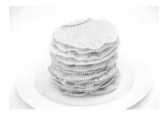

lamb keema kaleji

serves 4

This should be made well in advance to allow the flavour to fully open. There is so much goodness in this dish. The peppers and spices aid digestion balanced with calming yoghurt.

¼ cup vegetable oil

2 bay leaves

dash of sriracha

4-5cm cinnamon stick, broken into chunks

3-5 green cardamom pods

4 red onions, chopped

4 garlic cloves, crushed

4cm piece fresh ginger, peeled and chopped

2-3 small chillies, finely chopped

2 tsp turmeric

2 tsp ground cumin

2 tsp salt

50g tomato purée

1 tin chopped tomatoes

500g ground lamb

250g greek style yoghurt

juice of 1 lime

1-2 tsp garam masala

small bunch of coriander, chopped

Warm the oil, bay leaves, sriracha, cinnamon and cardamom in a large pan until the spices start to pop. Do not burn. Add the onions and garlic and cook without colour. Next, add the ginger, chillies, turmeric, cumin, salt, tomato purée and tomatoes and simmer for about 30 minutes. Add water to maintain a saucy consistency.

Next add the meat, stirring frequently to ensure a consistent texture. When the meat is cooked through, add the yoghurt and simmer for another few minutes. To finish, season with lime juice and garam masala and sprinkle with coriander. Serve hot with yoghurt and diced cucumber on chapattis.

Each portion provides 31g protein and 540kcals

nutrient	thumbs-up score
vitamin B6	>👍👍👍👍
vitamin B12	>👍👍👍👍
phosphorus	👍👍👍
sodium	👍👍👍
chloride	👍👍👍
protein	👍👍👍
vitamin C	👍👍
iodine	👍👍
iron	👍👍
protein	👍👍
zinc	👍👍
vitamin A (total retinol equivalents)	👍
niacin	👍
riboflavin	👍
thiamin	👍
calcium	👍
copper	👍
magnesium	👍
potassium	👍

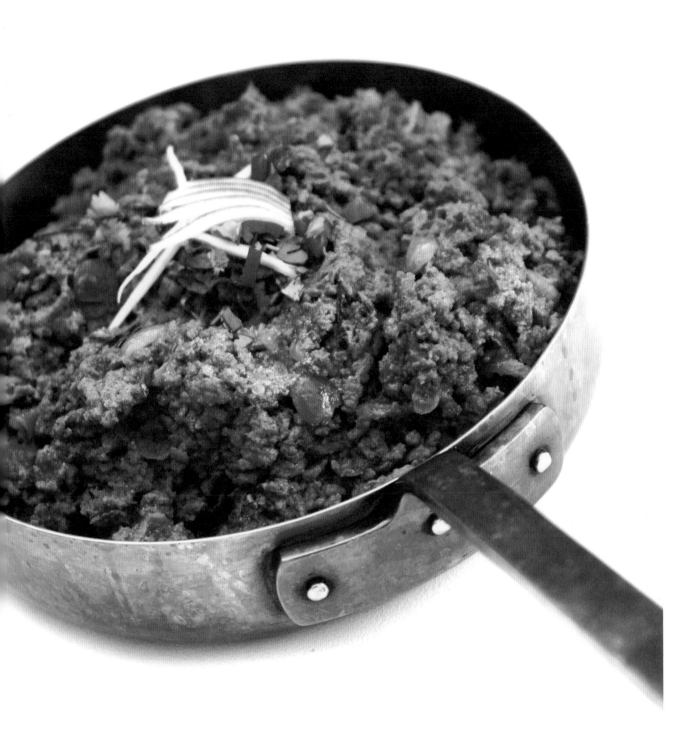

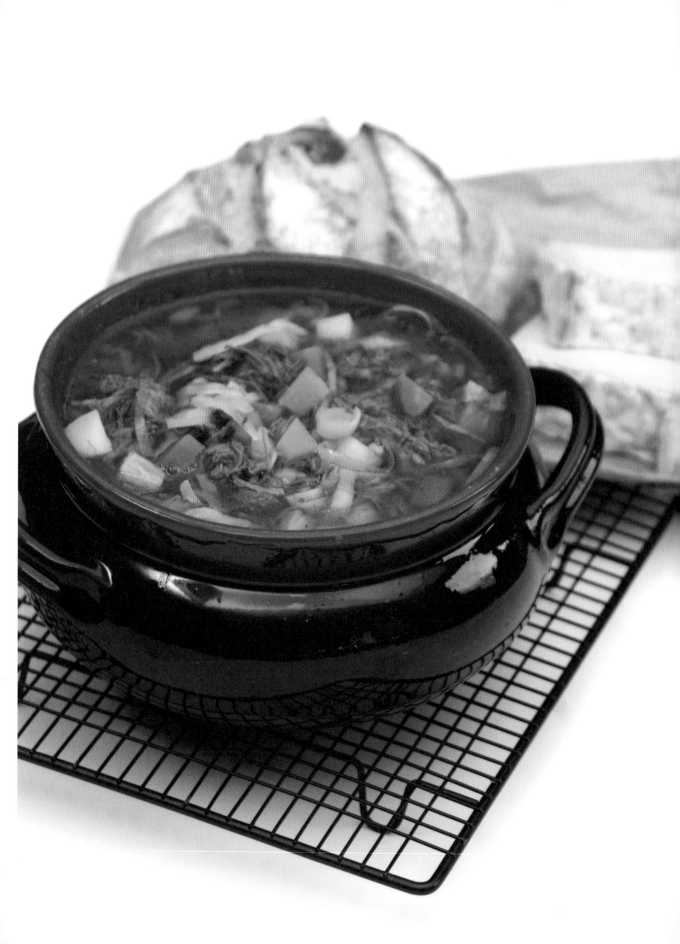

welsh cawl

serves 4

This is a showcase of winter veg and surprisingly light as the broth is not thickened. My Welsh neighbour Louise insists it should be served with a wedge of Caerphilly cheese and a chunk of wholegrain bread.

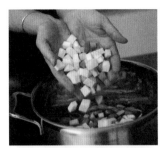

500g lamb shoulder
60ml sunflower oil
1 onion
2 carrots
½ swede
1 parsnip
½ small celeriac or 2 celery sticks
¼ small white cabbage, finely shredded
sprigs of parsley and thyme
2 ½ litres lamb stock
1 leek, white only
1 large potato, peeled
salt & pepper

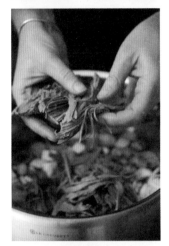

Cut the meat into 1 inch pieces, removing fat and sinew.

Peel and dice the root vegetables into uniform and small pieces. Clean the leek and finely chop this along with the onion and celeriac.

Next, on medium heat coat a large saucepan with oil then add the meat and brown. Remove the meat then add the onion and cook without colour. (Browning the onion will make it bitter).

Return the meat to the pan and add the onion, carrot, swede, parsnip, and celeriac. Mix well and cover with stock.

Bring to the boil and add the parsley and thyme. Simmer for about an hour, adding the potato and leek after 30 minutes and more stock or water if required. Simmer until the potatoes and leeks are soft. Season to taste and serve with cheese and bread.

Each portion provides 22g protein and 330kcals

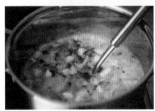

nutrient	thumbs-up score
sodium	>👍👍👍👍
chloride	>👍👍👍👍
vitamin B12	👍👍👍👍
vitamin B6	👍👍👍
vitamin C	👍👍
phosphorus	👍👍
protein	👍👍
zinc	👍👍
folate	👍
niacin	👍
thiamin	👍
copper	👍
potassium	👍

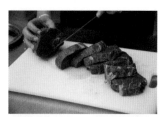

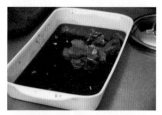

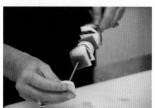

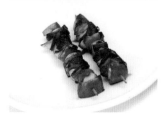

beef teriyaki brochettes
serves 4, 2 brochettes per person

This is a fun meal easy to prepare and serve and a great way to start the bbq season.

teriyaki marinade
120ml tamari soy
120ml mirin
2 tbsp sugar
juice of 1 lime
1 garlic clove, smashed
1 inch ginger, peeled and finely chopped
1 tbsp honey
½ tsp wasabi powder

1.75 kg beef fillet
2 large white onions
4 green peppers
16-20 medium closed cup mushrooms
8 bamboo skewers

marinade
Combine all ingredients in a saucepan, place on medium heat and bring to the boil and allow to simmer for 2-3 minutes. Be careful not to let the mixture boil too hard. Remove from heat and strain then allow to cool.

to build the brochettes
Cut the beef into 1½ inch cubes and cut the onions and peppers into 1½ inch squares. Wash and pat dry the mushrooms. Next spear the ingredients onto the skewers in rotating order starting with a pepper, onion, beef cube, onion, pepper, mushroom then repeat.

Place the brochettes in a shallow dish and cover with the marinade. Cover and place in refrigerator for at least 3 hours.

When ready to cook, preheat a bbq or skillet to high heat and sear on all sides then cook to medium rare to medium and serve hot.

Each portion provides 95g protein and 680kcal.

nutrient	thumbs-up score
vitamin B6	>👍👍👍👍
vitamin B12	>👍👍👍👍
vitamin C	>👍👍👍👍
phosphorus	>👍👍👍👍
protein	>👍👍👍👍
zinc	>👍👍👍👍
niacin	👍👍👍👍
riboflavin	👍👍👍👍
iron	👍👍👍👍
folate	👍👍
potassium	👍👍
selenium	👍👍
sodium	👍👍
chloride	👍👍
vitamin D	👍
thiamin	👍
copper	👍
iodine	👍
magnesium	👍

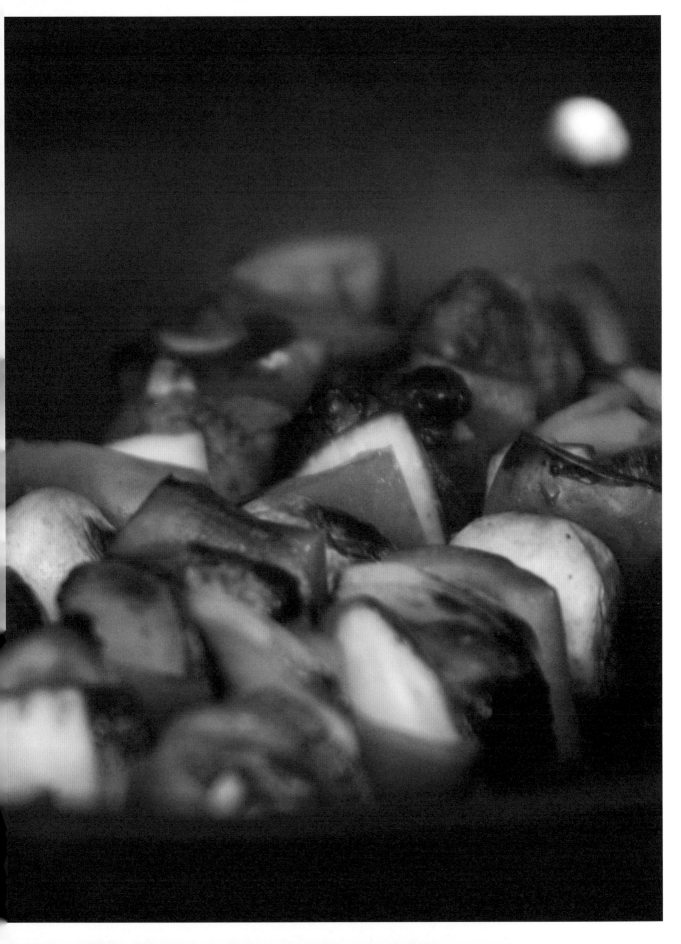

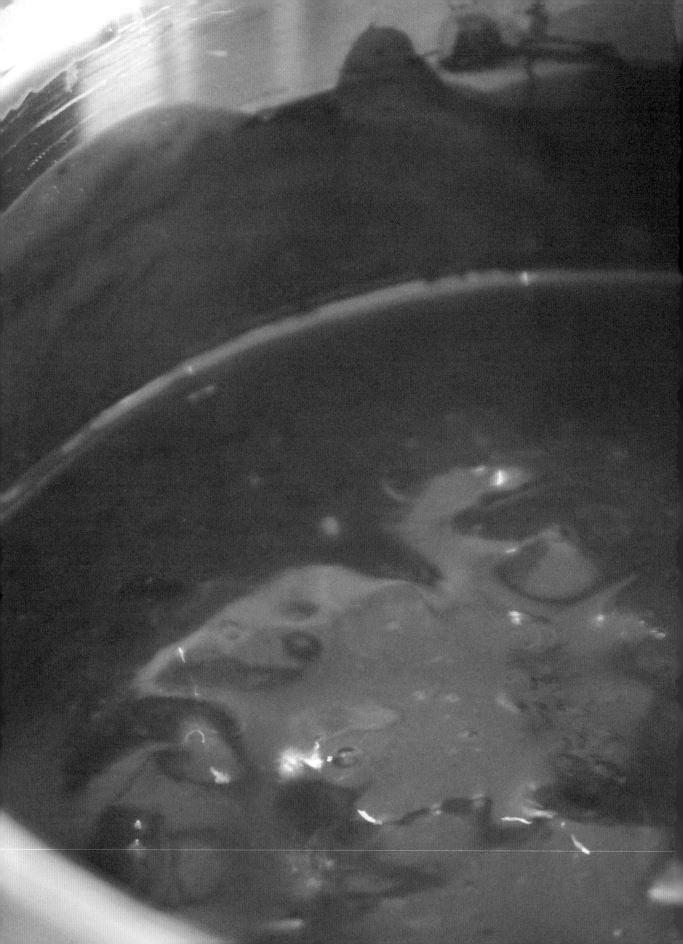

sweeties

sweeties

apple & rhubarb crumble 251

caramelised pears with cardamom & ginger &
    honey ice cream 252

plum frangipane tart 255

lemon loaf 256

baked apples & cinnamon ice cream 258

auntie winona's brownies 259

chocolate & beetroot tart 261

gin & tonic ice lollies 262

chocolate rum truffles 263

chocolate silk pie 264

pavlova 267

zabaglioni marsala with berries & biscotti 268

lemon posset 270

limoncello gelato 270

peppered pineapple with crème de cacao sauce &
    vanilla ice cream 271

champagne jelly 273

lemon tart 274

zucchini bread 277

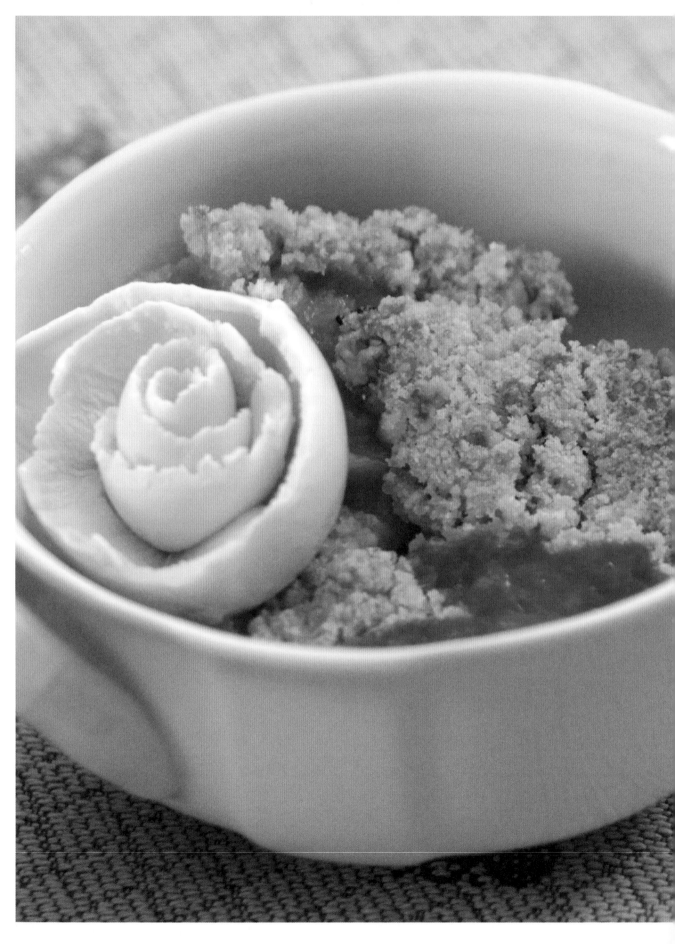

apple & rhubarb crumble

serves 4-6

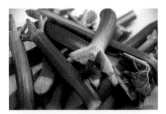

The delicious smell as this bakes is almost as good as the flavour. Though not really a nutritional heavyweight, it's a big bowl full of relaxation.

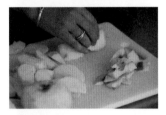

6 stalks rhubarb

120ml water

50ml caster sugar

3 cooking apples

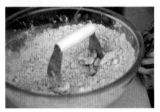

for the crumble

225g flour

100g demerara sugar

100g butter

1 tsp grated ginger, or powdered

Preheat oven to 160°Cf.

Trim and slice the rhubarb into 1 inch chunks and place in a baking tin. Sprinkle over the water and caster sugar and put in the oven to bake.

After about 30 minutes peel and slice the apples and add to the rhubarb. Bake for a further 30 minutes until cooked through and soft, then place in a deep buttered baking dish.

Mix together the crumble ingredients to an even but chunky consistency then sprinkle over the fruit. Bake for 40 minutes or until bubbly and golden brown. Serve with ice cream, warm custard or crème fraiche.

Each portion provides 4g protein and 350kcals

nutrient	thumbs-up score
vitamin B6	>👍 👍 👍 👍
vitamin C	👍 👍
vitamin A (total retinol equivalents)	👍
fibre (as non-starch polysaccharide)	👍

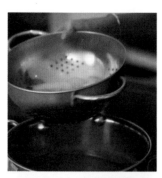

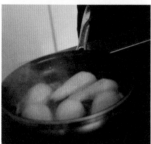

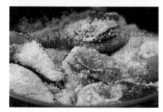

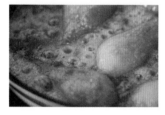

caramelised pears with cardamom & ginger & honey ice cream
serves 4

This is such a pretty pudding. The pears are sweet and tender and the ice cream is like a sweet gingery kiss.

500ml vanilla ice cream

150ml honey

250ml stem ginger in syrup, chopped

4 pears, not quite ripe conference are best

juice of 1 lemon

100g caster sugar

350g demerara sugar

1 tsp ground cardamom

Mix together the ice cream, honey and ginger and return to the freezer. Prepare well in advance, overnight is best.

Peel, halve and core the pears and poach in a pint of water with the caster sugar and half the lemon juice. Bring to the boil and simmer for a few minutes until tender but firm. Remove the pears and allow to cool.

Mix together the demerara sugar, cardamom and the rest of the lemon juice and leave for 30 minutes.

To serve, grill the poached pear halves until lightly coloured. Stir the sugar mixture over a medium heat until caramelised. Drizzle over the pears and serve with the ginger honey ice cream.

Each portion provides 6g protein and 795kcals

nutrient	thumbs-up score
vitamin B6	>👍👍👍👍
vitamin B12	👍👍
vitamin C	👍
riboflavin	👍
calcium	👍
copper	👍
fibre (as non-starch polysaccharide)	👍
iodine	👍
phosphorous	👍

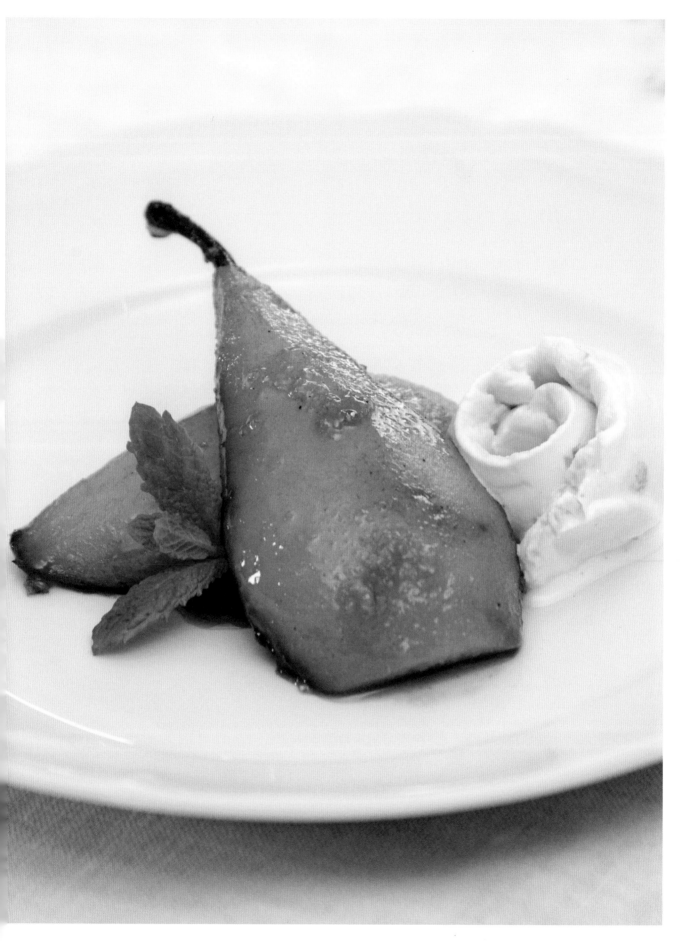

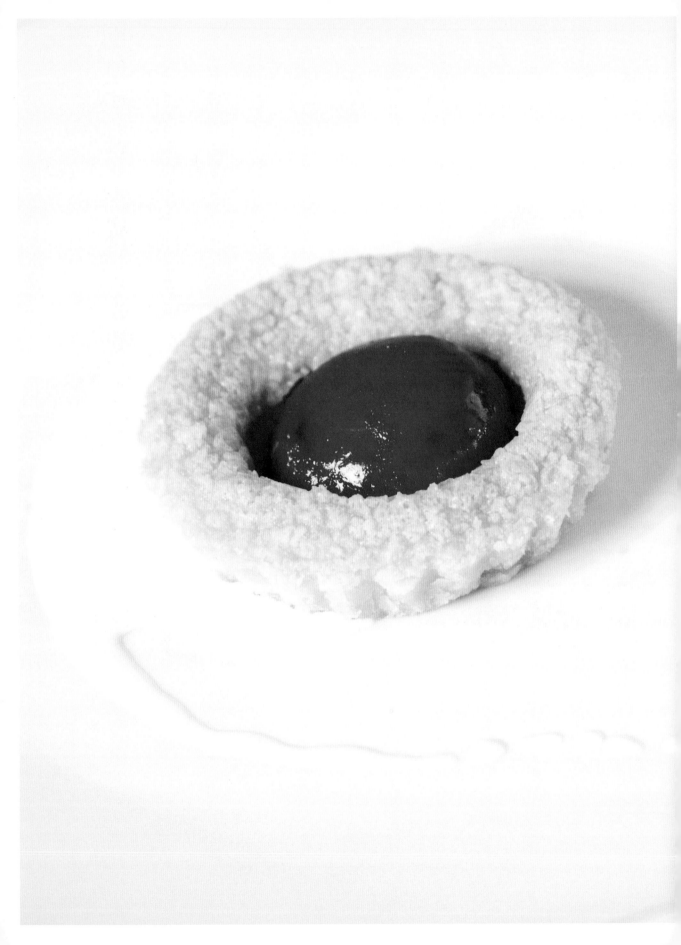

plum frangipane tart
yields 1 9inch tart or use ½ plum per individual tart

There is a bit more to this luscious tart than it seems. Its packed with vitamins and other nutrients and the plums pack a flavour wallop.

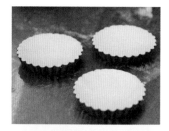

500g ready-made puff pastry
100g butter
225g ground almonds
5 eggs
250ml single cream
225g golden caster sugar
6-15 plums depending on size, halved and stoned
2 tbsp demerara sugar

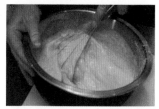

Preheat oven to 180°Cf.

Prepare the puff pastry in a loose-bottomed tart tin or individual tartlets. Chill for 30 minutes then blind bake, remove from the oven and allow to cool.

Melt the butter in a saucepan then whisk in the almonds, eggs, cream and sugar until smooth. Pour into the pastry case.

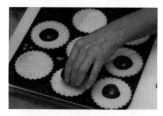

Arrange the plums cut-side down, pushing them into the mixture. They should fit fairly close together or use ½ plum per tartlet. Sprinkle with the sugar and bake for 25-30 minutes or until the filling is just set and the plums are cooked. (The tartlets should take about half the time so keep an eye on them.)

Each portion provides 20g protein and 910kcals

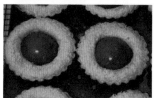

nutrient	thumbs-up score
vitamin B12	> 👍👍👍
vitamin A (total retinol equivalents)	👍👍👍
vitamin B6	👍👍👍
phosphorus	👍👍👍
riboflavin	👍👍
copper	👍👍
magnesium	👍👍
folate	👍
thiamin	👍
calcium	👍
fibre (as non-starch polysaccharide)	👍
iodine	👍
iron	👍
potassium	👍
protein	👍
sodium	👍
chloride	👍
zinc	👍

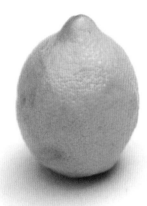

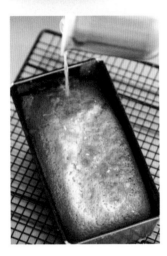

lemon loaf
yields 1 loaf

My friends call this 'the luscious lemon loaf'. That says it all. If you want to zest it up, use extra lemon juice in the glaze.

100g butter

225g caster sugar

2 eggs

120ml milk

350g flour

1 tsp baking powder

½ tsp salt

glaze
zest and juice of 1 lemon

50g caster sugar

Preheat oven to 170°Cf.

Mix together the butter, sugar, eggs and milk in one bowl. In another bowl, combine the flour, baking powder and salt. Mix together the contents of the two bowls to make a smooth batter. Pour into a greased and floured loaf pan and bake for 60 minutes or until a toothpick comes out clean.

As soon as the loaf comes out of the oven, heat the lemon juice, lemon zest and sugar in a saucepan, bring to a boil without colouring and drizzle over the loaf. Allow to cool before serving.

Each portion provides 4g protein and 300kcals

nutrient	thumbs-up score
vitamin B6	> 👍👍👍👍
vitamin A (total retinol equivalents)	👍
phosphorus	👍
sodium	👍
chloride	👍

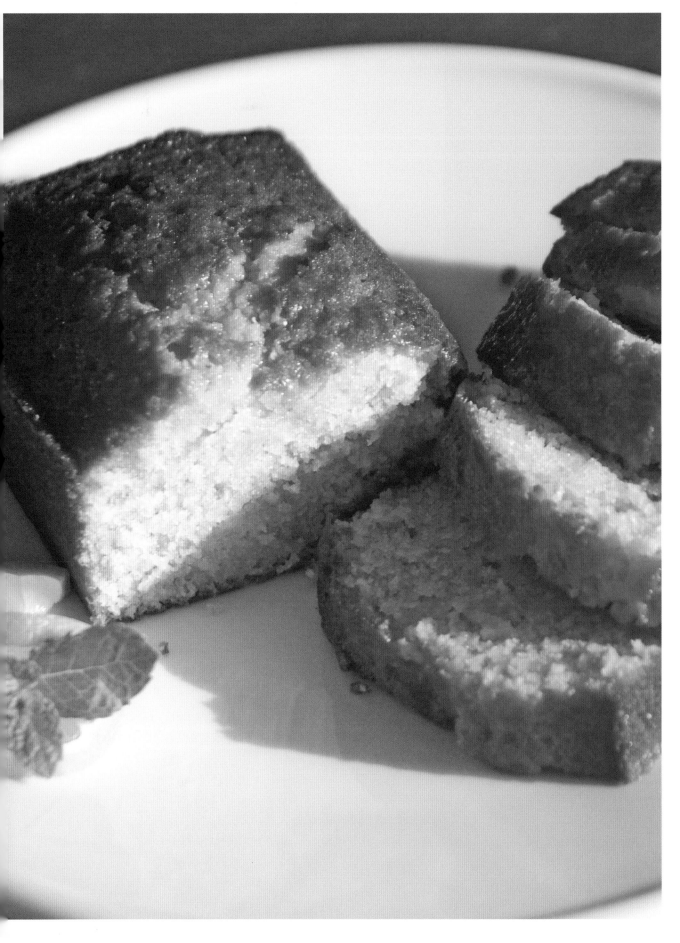

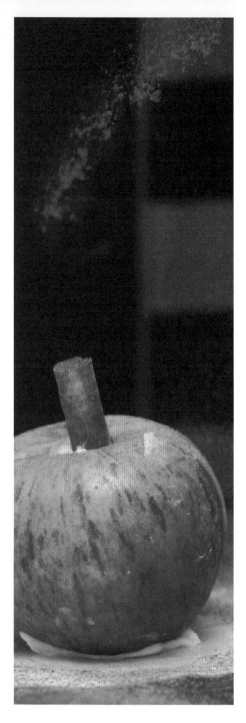

baked apples & cinnamon ice cream

serves 4, 1 apple per person

Comfort food! This is great on a cool winter evening.

apples

4 apples, tart and firm such as braeburn or mackintosh

butter

cinnamon sticks

cinnamon ice cream

225ml milk

1 cinnamon stick

3 egg yolks

100g sugar

1 tsp ground cinnamon

450ml whipping or double cream

Prepare the ice cream well in advance. At least 3 hours. Put the milk in a pan with the cinnamon stick and bring to the boil. In a separate bowl, whisk together the egg yolks, sugar and ground cinnamon. Discard the cinnamon stick, then strain the hot milk over the yolks, whisking continuously. (For a quick cheat add ground cinnamon and a bit of brown sugar to vanilla ice cream).

Pour the mixture into a well-chilled bowl. Freeze for 1½ hours or until starting to freeze. Stir well, then repeat the process twice more until the mixture is smooth. Transfer to a sealed container and keep frozen until ready to serve.

Preheat oven to 170°Cf.

Cut individual sheets of tin foil large enough to wrap each apple and smear with soft butter.

Core the apples and insert a cinnamon stick. Place on the buttered foil and dust with ground cinnamon. Wrap and seal to create a loose parcel. Bake for 15-20 minutes. Serve immediately with cinnamon ice cream.

Each portion provides 7g protein and 700kcals

nutrient	thumbs-up score
vitamin B6	>👍👍👍👍
vitamin B12	>👍👍👍👍
vitamin A (total retinol equivalents)	👍👍👍👍
riboflavin	👍
calcium	👍
iodine	👍
phosphorus	👍

auntie winona's brownies
yields 1, 9inch square tin

This recipe is an Ericson family classic. They are so chocolatey and irresistible. Bet you can't stop at one!

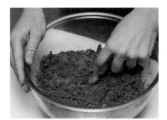

½ cup butter, softened
1 cup confectioners (icing) sugar
½ cup cocoa (add a splash of hot water for easy mixing)
2 eggs
½ cup flour
1 tsp vanilla extract
pinch of table salt

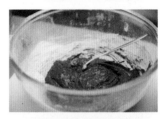

Preheat oven to 180°Cf.

Cream the butter, sugar and cocoa. Add the rest of the ingredients and mix until thoroughly blended and creamy. The batter should be thick and smooth. Pour into a 9 x 9in greased cake tin and bake for 20-30 minutes or until a toothpick comes out clean.

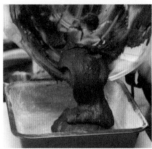

icing
2 tbsp butter
2 tbsp cocoa
2 cups icing sugar
1 tsp vanilla extract
pinch of salt

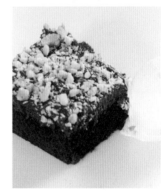

Put all the ingredients in a bowl and whip together until smooth. Ice the brownies while still warm then sprinkle with a layer of chopped walnuts. Serve plain or with vanilla ice cream.

Each portion provides 10g protein and 1230kcals

nutrient	thumbs-up score
vitamin A (total retinol equivalents)	👍👍👍👍
copper	👍👍👍
sodium	👍👍👍
chloride	👍👍
vitamin B6	👍👍
phosphorus	👍👍
iodine	👍
iron	👍
magnesium	👍
zinc	👍

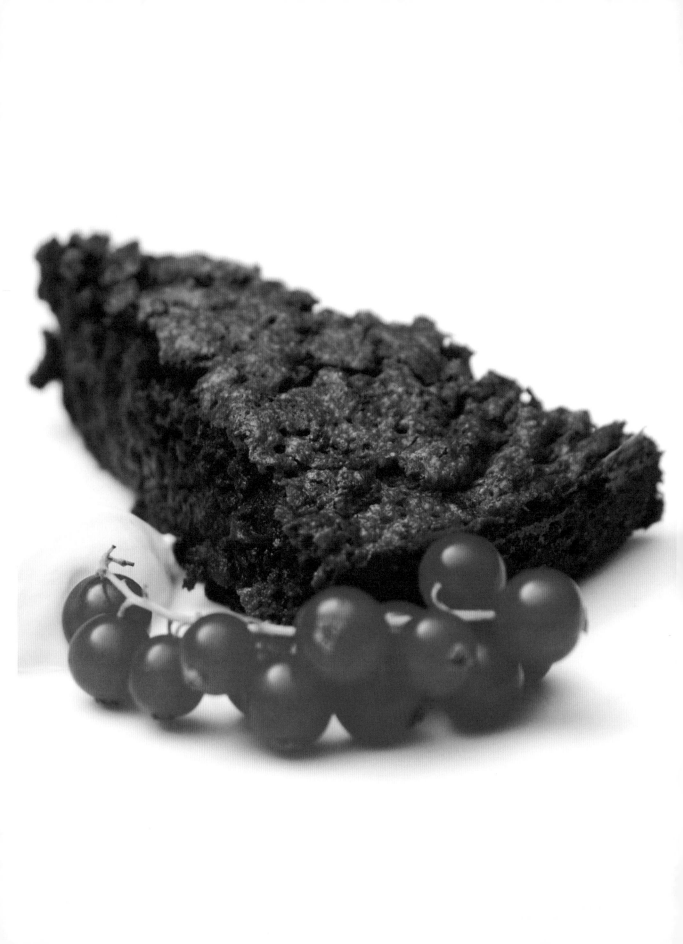

chocolate & beetroot tart
yields 1, 9inch tart

This is a clever way to get one of your best friends, beetroot, into the mix (literally). The natural sugar of the beetroot has an earthier flavour and also gives this tart a very moist texture. If you don't tell anyone they won't notice!

100g dark chocolate

100g butter, melted

300g light brown sugar

3 eggs

225g flour

50g dry cocoa

¼ tsp salt

250g beetroot, cooked, peeled and grated

Preheat oven to 180°Cf.

Line a 9 inch loose-bottomed cake tin with parchment.

Melt 75g of the chocolate over simmering water. Finely chop the rest.

Mix together the butter, sugar and eggs until the sugar is completely dissolved. Stir in the melted chocolate. Sift together the flour, cocoa and salt, then fold into the chocolate mixture.

Finally, stir in the beetroot and chopped chocolate. Pour into the cake tin and bake for about 20-25 minutes or until a toothpick comes out almost clean.

Allow to cool for 5 minutes, then remove from the tin. Serve with a tablespoon of crème fraiche.

Each portion provides 16g protein and 1070kcals

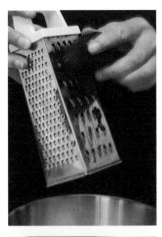

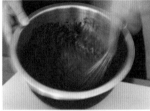

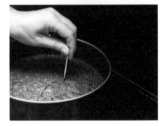

nutrient	thumbs-up score
vitamin A (total retinol equivalents)	👍👍👍
vitamin B12	👍👍👍
copper	👍👍👍
phosphorus	👍👍👍
vitamin B6	👍👍
iron	👍👍
magnesium	👍👍
sodium	👍👍
chloride	👍
folate	👍
riboflavin	👍
calcium	👍
fibre (non-starch polysaccaride)	👍
iodine	👍
potassium	👍
protein	👍
zinc	👍

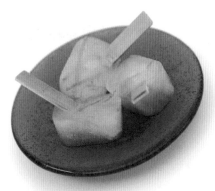

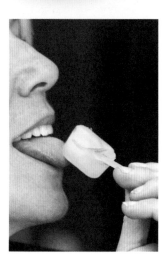

gin & tonic ice lollies
makes 6 large or 8 small

This is a number one hit in Marie Curie Cancer Care Centres. No protein but a real morale booster and posh way to help with dry mouth and nausea and to stimulate appetite. Bring 'em on!

6 tbsp gin (or vodka)*

375ml sugar syrup (250g caster sugar)

375ml tonic water

1 lime (or lemon)

To make the sugar syrup, bring 250g caster sugar and 250ml water to the boil to completely dissolve the sugar and allow to cool.

Zest and juice the lime then strain the juice. Mix together the gin, sugar syrup, tonic water and juice. Pour into lolly moulds, allowing 1cm clearance at the top and freeze overnight.

One lolly provides 0 protein and 359kcals

* If you want the flavour but not the alcohol you can infuse the sugar syrup by heating it with a few juniper berries.

nutrient   thumbs-up score

sorry, we couldn't analyse this recipe, it only gets a thumbs-up for fun!   >👍👍👍👍

chocolate rum truffles
yields 25-30 truffles

People often crave chocolate when in treatment. These are more-ish with a capital M. What's so great is that they are a great small portion and soft so easy to eat.

300ml double cream

300g dark chocolate, chopped, 75% cocoa solids

50-60 ml navy or spiced rum

1 tsp salt

cocoa powder

Place the cream in a pan over a medium heat and bring up to a simmer.

Melt the chocolate in a large bowl over a saucepan of simmering water.

When the cream is simmering, remove the pan from the heat, add the salt, and add to the melted chocolate a third at a time, making sure that the cream is thoroughly incorporated after each addition. Allow to cool slightly.

Pour the chocolate mixture into a bowl and leave to stand at room temperature for 4 hours, then place in the fridge for 5-6 hours or until set. This irresistible concoction is called ganache.

Using a teaspoon, scoop spoon-sized chunks of the ganache onto a plate loaded with cocoa. Generously coat your hands with cocoa then roll the chunks in cocoa powder. Chill for at least an hour before serving. If you can wait that long.

Each portion provides 3g protein and 300kcals
(analysed 5 truffles per portion)

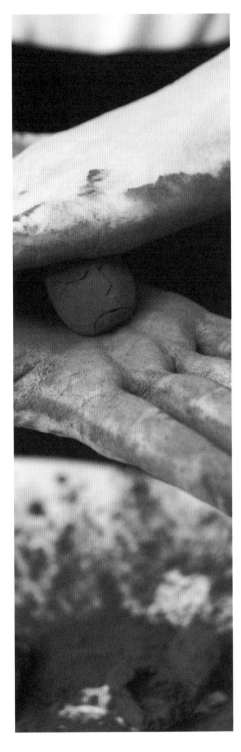

nutrient	thumbs-up score
vitamin A (total retinol equivalents)	👍👍👍
vitamin B12	👍
copper	👍
sodium	👍
chloride	👍

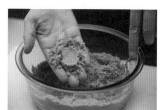

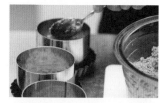

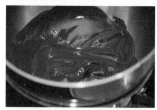

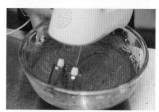

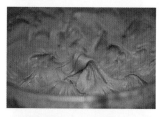

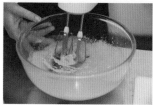

chocolate silk pie
yields 1, 9inch pie

Chocolate Silk Pie, even the name has a bit of 'come hither' about it. If you fancy smooth and elegant chocolate this is just the ticket.

crust
275g graham or digestive biscuit crumbs

50g butter

filling
150g butter, softened

2 tsp pure vanilla

200g sugar

90g baking chocolate, unsweetened

3 large eggs

topping
150g whipping cream

chocolate shavings

Prepare the crust by melting the butter and stirring in the biscuit crumbs. Press into a 9inch spring form pan or individual moulds and chill.

To make the filling, cream the butter and vanilla in a large mixing bowl with a hand mixer at medium to high speed for about 1 minute. Gradually add the sugar while continuing to beat until the mixture is light and fluffy and not granular – this will take several minutes and is essential to the success of the recipe.

Melt the chocolate in bowl over a pan of boiling water. Add to the butter mixture beating until the chocolate is well blended and the mixture is smooth and creamy.

Finally, add the eggs one at a time, beating in each before adding the next until the mixture is light and fluffy. Pour the filling into the crust, smooth the top and then chill for several hours until set. When set top with whipped cream and chocolate shavings.

Each portion provides 39g protein and 471kcals

nutrient	thumbs-up score
vitamin B6	👍👍👍
vitamin A (total retinol equivalents)	👍👍
vitamin B12	👍👍
sodium	👍
chloride	👍

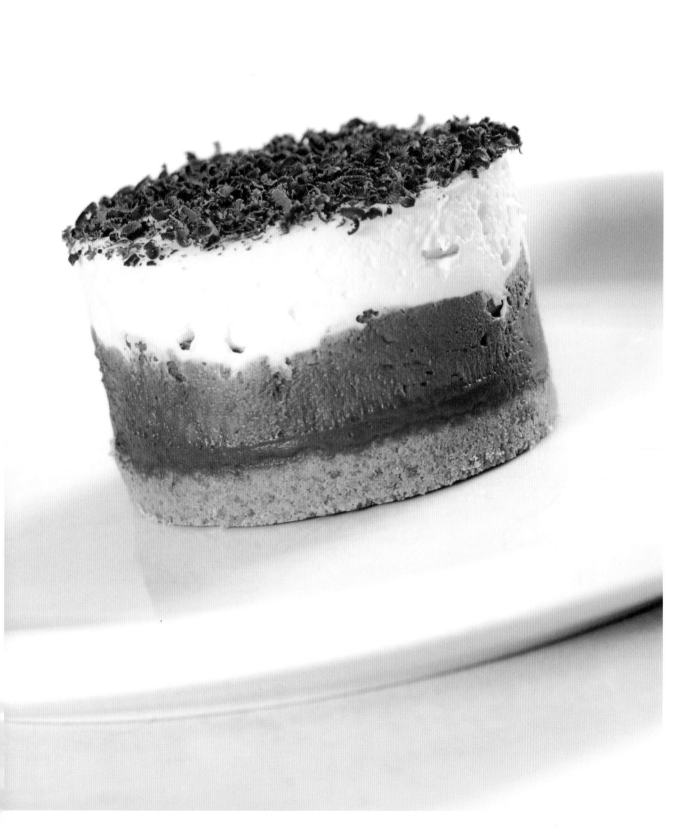

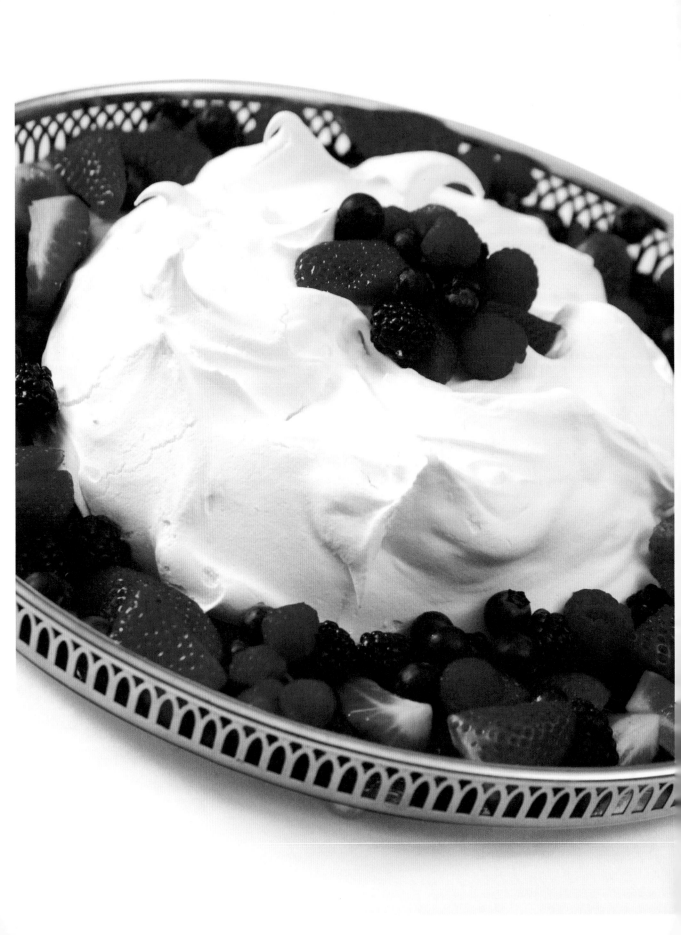

pavlova

serves 8

When you say 'pavlova', the universal response is a lip smacking. You get to eat this pudding twice, first with your eyes!

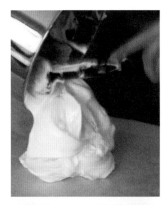

4 large egg whites
200g caster sugar
200g of fresh berries or other seasonal fruit
200ml whipping cream
30g fresh ginger, grated (optional)

Preheat oven to 150°Cf.

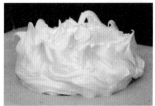

Chill a glass bowl and cover a baking tray with a sheet of parchment. Also, make sure all utensils are clean and dry, as egg whites are very sensitive and react to even small amounts of oil and foods.

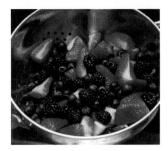

In the chilled bowl beat the egg whites to medium soft peaks with an electric mixer at high speed, scraping the sides frequently. Reduce speed to low and slowly add the sugar. Switch back to high speed for 1 minute. The peaks should be stiff.

Heap the mixture onto the parchment and use a spoon to form peaks. Be careful not to flatten. Place in the middle of the oven, turn the heat down to 100°Cf and bake for 1 hour. Do not open the oven door as the pavlova will collapse. Turn the oven off and let the pavlova rest until completely cool.

Serve with fruit and whipped cream. To add a hint of spice, grate a little fresh ginger into the fruit just before serving.

Each portion provides 5g protein and 415kcals

nutrient	thumbs-up score
vitamin B6	👍👍👍👍
vitamin C	👍👍
vitamin A (total retinol equivalents)	👍

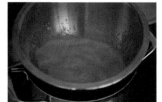
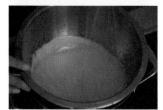
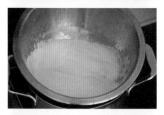
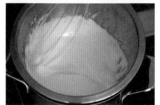
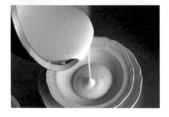

zabaglione marsala with berries & biscotti

serves 4

This pudding is like eating air. It's light, smooth and rich at the same time. It may not win any awards for its nutritional value, but it's easy to make and a lovely way to refresh challenged tastebuds.

3 egg yolks
40g caster sugar
40ml white wine
25ml marsala wine

Mix all of the ingredients together in a large stainless steel bowl then place over a saucepan of boiling water. Whisk until foaming and ribbons form. Continue whisking for 1 minute, then pour into warmed glasses. Serve immediately with fresh fruit and biscotti.

The ribbon stage in whisking is specific. As you lift the whisk from the cream, it will fall back upon itself but should leave a trail or ribbon across the surface. This ribbon should not sink back in but hold firm.

biscotti

125g caster sugar
40g flour
50g butter, softened
65g flaked almonds
juice and zest of 1 orange
a mixture of fresh berries to garnish

Preheat oven to 180°Cf.

Mix all of the ingredients together in a bowl. Using a tablespoon, create rounds on a non-stick baking sheet or paper. Allow for spreading between each round. Bake until golden brown, then remove and drape each soft biscuit over a rolling pin and allow to cool. Store in an airtight container.

Don't be surprised if the biscotti are a bit chewier than store bought, they're still great.

Each portion provides 7g protein and 470kcals

nutrient	thumbs-up score
vitamin B12	👍👍👍
vitamin A (total retinol equivalents)	👍
vitamin C	👍
copper	👍
iron	👍

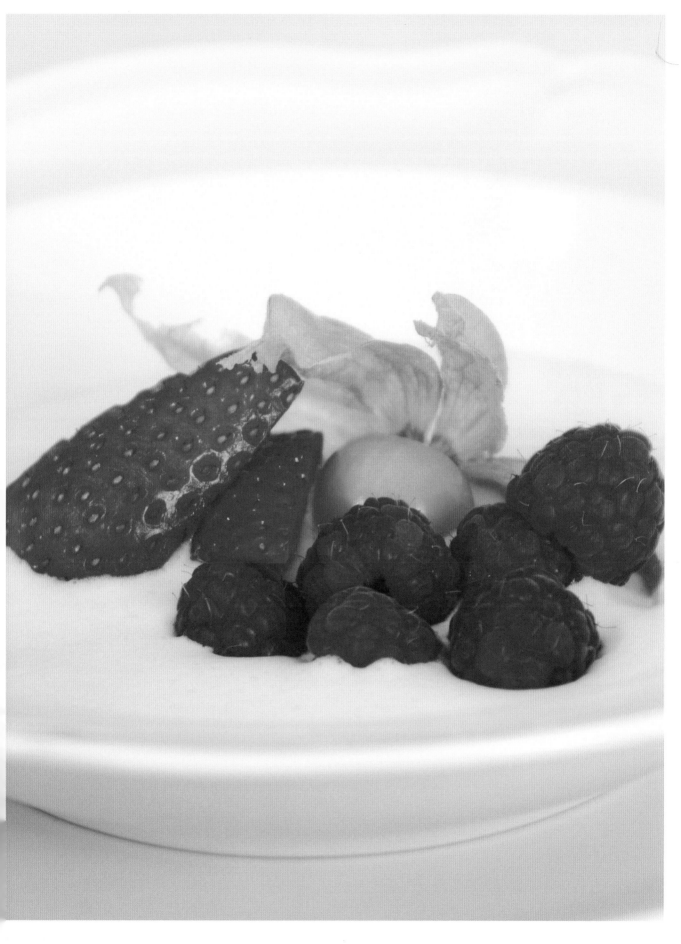

nutrient	thumbs-up score
vitamin A (total retinol equivalents)	>👍👍👍👍
riboflavin	👍
iodine	👍

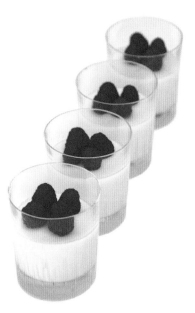

lemon posset

serves 4

This is such a wee dainty pudding but it packs a wallop. It's not a nutritional giant, it's so fresh and palette cleansing and the creamy lemon cuts through plastic mouth and is easy to swallow.

600ml double cream

150g granulated sugar

juice and zest of 2 lemons

fresh raspberries for garnish

Over low heat bring the cream and sugar just to the boil and simmer for 3 minutes. The sugar should be completely dissolved. Whisk in the lemon juice and zest and pour into glasses and chill until ready to serve.

Be careful when zesting the lemon to take only the yellow of the skin, the white is bitter.

Each portion provides 3g protein and 890kcals

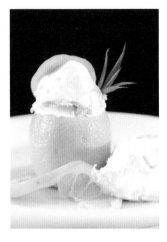

limoncello gelato

I get asked for this more than any other dessert. It's a little tastebud tingling jewel. A vitamin best friend, creamy cool texture the limoncello gives it mouth-watering flavour. It is soothing on the throat as well.

juice and zest of 3 large lemons

190g icing sugar

450ml double cream

3 tbsp limoncello, frozen

Place the lemon zest and juice in a bowl. Add the icing sugar, stir to combine and leave for 30 minutes.

Whip the cream and limoncello to soft peaks, then add the lemon and sugar mixture and whip together. Freeze overnight. Spoon the mixture into hollowed lemon halves to serve.

Each portion provides 2g protein and 790kcals

nutrient	thumbs-up score
vitamin A (total retinol requirements)	>👍👍👍👍
vitamin B6	>👍👍👍👍
vitamin B6	>👍👍👍👍
vitamin B12	👍👍
iodine	👍

peppered pineapple with crème de cacao sauce & vanilla ice cream
serves 1 pineapple ring per person

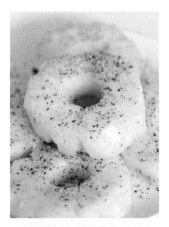

This pudding is festive and fun all year round. Pineapple and pepper make a tantalising pair. Try grilling the pineapple on the bbq.

100g caster sugar

25ml butter

juice and zest of 1 orange

juice and zest of 1 lemon

50ml crème de cacao

25ml brown butter*

1 whole pineapple

freshly cracked black pepper

4 scoops vanilla ice cream

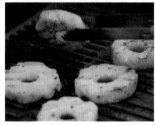

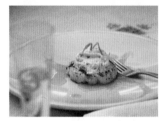

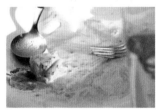

Melt the sugar together with a knob of butter until brown, then add the orange and lemon zest and juice and crème de cacao. Simmer briefly, stir in the brown butter and keep warm.

Cut off the top and bottom of the pineapple and stand up on a board. A bread knife is a good tool for this. Notice that the eyes run down in columns. Take off the skin in vertical slices, with a column of eyes in the centre, just deep enough to remove them. Follow the shape of the fruit. Use a paring knife to remove any leftover eyes, then cut in 1 inch thick slices. If the core is a bit hard, remove it.

Crack black pepper on both sides of the slices then fry in a knob of butter until lightly coloured. Season with a bit more pepper. Place on a plate and drizzle with the fruity syrup. Serve with a scoop of vanilla ice cream.

Each portion provides 3g protein and 470kcals

*see *the basics*, page 280

nutrient	thumbs-up score
vitamin B6	👍👍👍👍
vitamin C	👍👍👍👍
vitamin A (total retinol equivalents)	👍
vitamin B12	👍
riboflavin	👍
thiamin	👍
copper	👍

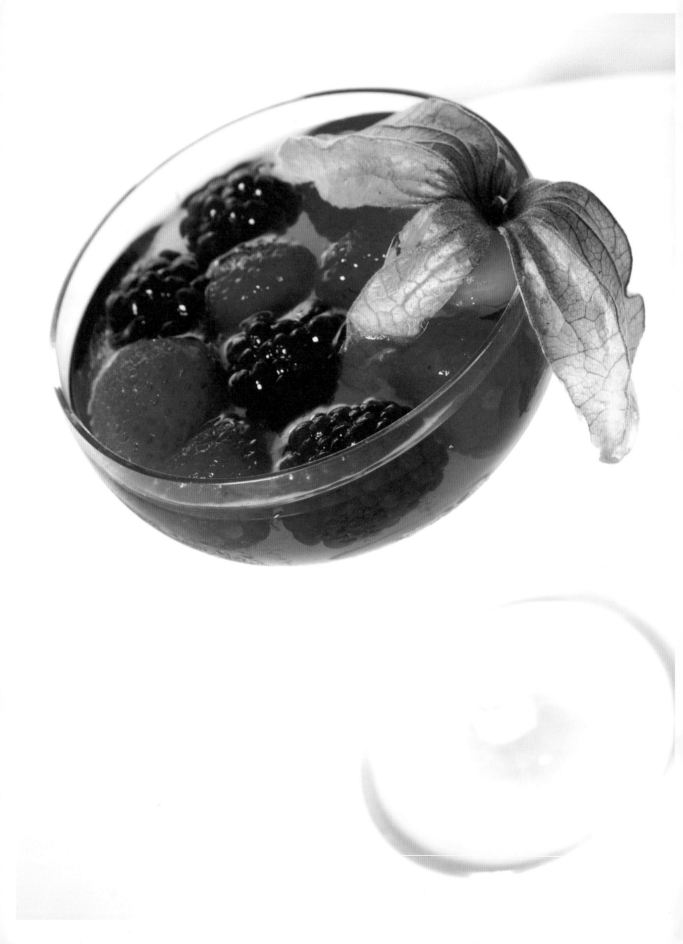

champagne jelly

serves 4

Like most jellies the greatest benefit comes from the cool texture soothing plastic or metal mouth. It's a playful dessert, easy to prepare and serve.

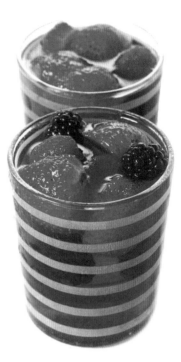

600ml champagne, less expensive fizz is fine
120g sugar
8 sheets, 20g leaf gelatine
a handful of fresh berries
300ml whipping cream for garnish

Place 4 jelly moulds or glasses into fridge to chill.

Place the gelatine leaves in cold water to allow to soften. Then pour the champagne into a saucepan on medium heat and add the sugar stirring constantly until sugar is fully dissolved. Do not allow the mixture to boil. Remove the gelatine from the water and add to the champagne mixture and whisk until completely dissolved. Remove from heat. Pour into chilled champagne glasses and arrange fruit on top. Place back in the fridge for several hours until firmly set.

For a more stylish presentation use jelly moulds. Remove moulds from fridge and add a shallow layer of jelly mixture then arrange the fruit. Place back in the fridge and allow to set. Cover with more jelly and repeat the process for as many layers as desired. As you wait for each layer to set keep the champagne mixture warm and in a liquid state. To serve turn the jellies onto serving plates and garnish with fresh fruit and whipped cream.

Each portion provides 6g protein and 540kcals

nutrient	thumbs-up score
vitamin B6	👍👍👍👍
vitamin C	👍👍👍
vitamin A (total retinol equivalents)	👍👍

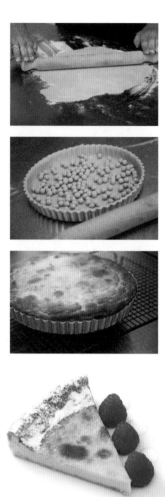

lemon tart
yields 1, 9inch tart

Lemon tart always brings a mouth-watering smile. It's like sunshine on a plate. It's a little vitamin booster as well.

short pastry, store bought is fine
5 eggs
150g caster sugar
150ml whipping cream
juice and zest of 2 lemons
juice of 1 orange
25g icing sugar
180g crème fraiche

Preheat oven to 160°Cf.

To prepare the crust follow packet instructions. Line a 9 inch tart tin and blind bake following the packet instructions and set aside to cool.

In a chilled glass bowl, whisk the eggs and caster sugar together until mixed, then add the whipping cream, lemon zest, lemon and orange juice and beat until smooth (but not frothy). Take care not to introduce too much air into the mixture.

Place the crust on a baking sheet positioned near the oven and pour in the mixture. Bake for approximately 30 minutes or until just done. The centre should spring to the touch. Do not allow the filling to brown. Dust with icing sugar and serve with a dollop of crème fraiche.

Each portion provides 10g protein and 850kcals

nutrient	thumbs-up score
vitamin A (total retinol equivalents)	👍👍👍👍
vitamin B12	👍👍👍
vitamin B6	👍👍👍
vitamin C	👍
riboflavin	👍
iodine	👍
iron	👍
phosphorus	👍
sodium	👍
chloride	👍

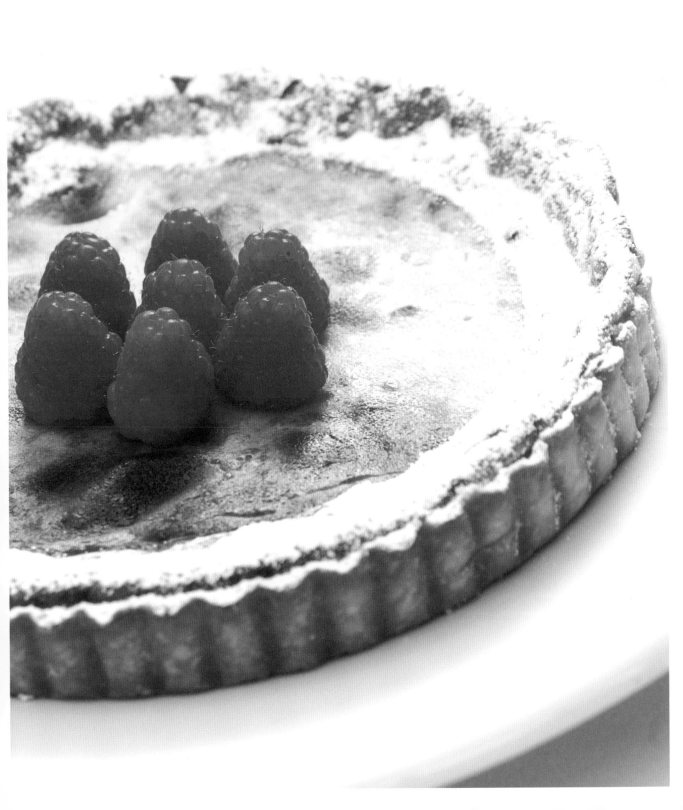

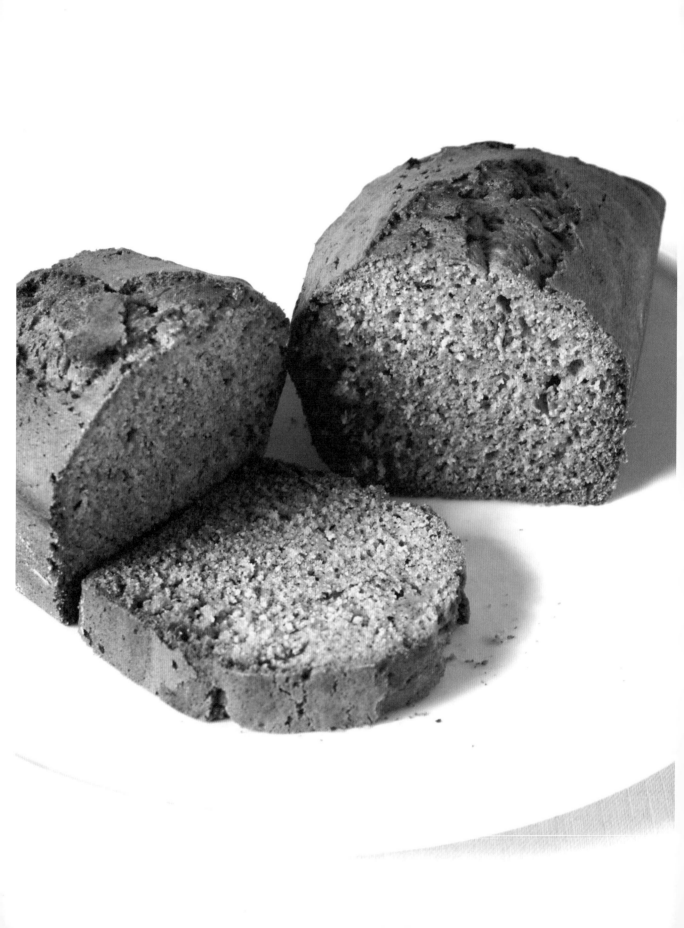

zucchini bread
yields 1 loaf, 8 slices

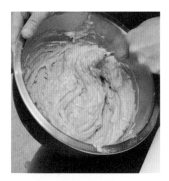

This recipe came from Italy so I haven't called it 'courgette bread.' It's more a coffee cake than a pudding with bags of flavour. It's simply scrumptious just out of the oven with lashings of butter or cream cheese.

2 eggs

½ cup sunflower or other light vegetable oil

1 cup granulated sugar

1 cup unpeeled zucchini, grated

1 tsp vanilla extract

2 cups flour

1 tsp baking powder

1 tsp baking soda

½ tsp salt

1 tsp cinnamon

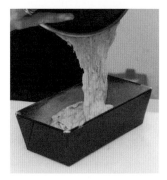

Preheat the oven to 180°Cf.

In a large mixing bowl beat the eggs until light and frothy, then add the oil, sugar and beat until smooth. Add the zucchini and vanilla extract.

In another bowl combine the flour, baking powder, soda, salt and cinnamon. Fold in the zucchini mixture until fully combined. Pour into a greased loaf pan and bake for 50-60 minutes or until a toothpick comes out clean.

It's delicious straight out of the oven with lashings of butter.

Each portion provides 5g protein and 370kcals

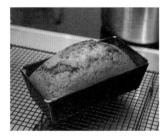

nutrient	thumbs-up score
vitamin B6	👍👍👍👍
vitamin B12	👍
iron	👍
potassium	👍

for our international friends

conversions

Liquid measures		Solid measures		Linear measures	
15ml	½ fl oz	5g	$^1/_8$ oz	3mm	$^1/_8$ inch
20ml	¾ fl oz	10g	¼ oz	5mm	¼ inch
25ml	1 fl oz	15g	½ oz	1cm	½ inch
35ml	1¼ fl oz	20g	¾ oz	2cm	¾ inch
40ml	1½ fl oz	25g	1 oz	2.5cm	1 inch
50ml	2 fl oz	40g	1½ oz	3cm	1 $^1/_8$ inch
60ml	2¼ fl oz	50g	2 oz	4cm	1 ½ inch
65ml	2½ fl oz	65g	2 ½ oz	4.5cm	1 ¼ inch
85ml	3 fl oz	75g	3 oz	5cm	2 inches
100ml	3½ fl oz	90g	3½ oz	6cm	2 ½ inches
120ml	4 fl oz	100g	4 oz (¼ lb)	7.5cm	3 inches
150ml	5 fl oz (¼ pint)	120g	4½ oz	9cm	3½ inches
175ml	6 fl oz	135g	4¾ oz	10cm	4 inches
200ml	7 fl oz	150g	5 oz	13cm	5 inches
250ml	8 fl oz	165g	5½ oz	15cm	6 inches
275ml	9 fl oz	175g	6 oz	18cm	7 inches
300ml	10 fl oz (½ pint)	185g	6½ oz	20cm	8 inches
325ml	11 fl oz	200g	7 oz	23cm	9 inches
350ml	12 fl oz	215g	7½ oz	25cm	10 inches
375ml	13 fl oz	225g	8 oz (½ lb)	28cm	11 inches
400ml	14 fl oz	250g	9 oz	30cm	12 inches (1 ft)
450ml	15 fl oz (¾ pint)	275g	10 oz		
475ml	16 fl oz	300g	11 oz		
500ml	17 fl oz	350g	12 oz (¾ lb)		
550ml	18 fl oz	375g	13 oz		
575ml	19 fl oz	400g	14 oz		
600ml	20 fl oz (1 pint)	425g	15 oz		
750ml	1¼ pints	450g	16 oz (1 lb)		
900ml	1½ pints	550g	1¼ lb		
1 ltr	1¾ pints	750g	1½ lb		
1.2 ltr	2 pints	1kg	2¼ lb		
1.25 ltr	2¼ pints	1.25kg	2½ lb		
1.5 ltr	2½ pints	1.5kg	3½ lb		
1.6 ltr	2¾ pints	1.75kg	4 lb		
1.75 ltr	3 pints	2kg	4½ lb		
2 ltr	3½ pints	2.25 g	5 lb		

Liquid measures

2.25 ltr	4 pints
2.5 ltr	4½ pints
2.75 ltr	5 pints
3.4 ltr	6 pints
3.9 ltr	7 pints
4.5 ltr	8 pints
5 ltr	9 pints

Solid measures

2.5 kg	5½ lb
2.75 kg	6 lb
3 kg	7 lb
3.5 kg	8 lb
4 kg	9 lb
4.5 kg	10 lb
5 kg	11 lb
5.5 kg	12 lb

Oven temperatures

Gas	C	C fan	F	Oven Temp
¼	110	90	225	very cool
½	120	100	250	very cool
1	140	120	275	cool or slow
2	150	130	300	cool or slow
3	160	140	325	warm
4	180	160	350	moderate
5	190	170	375	medium hot
6	200	180	400	fairly hot
7	220	200	425	hot
8	230	210	450	very hot
9	240	220	275	very hot

the basics
These are some of the principles we follow and a few traditional methods

blind-bake
Partially baking a pastry crust before filling it ensures it won't go soggy. Line the crust with parchment and fill with ceramic baking beans (or uncooked beans or rice) and place in a medium oven for about 5-8 minutes. Do not allow to turn colour. Remove the beans and parchment.

boiling pasta
When using dry pasta, generously salt the water, approximately 1 tbsp per litre of water. When the pasta is ready, strain and rinse thoroughly in cold water to stop the cooking process and remove excess starch. If the pasta is going to be standing for a time before being used add a small amount of olive oil to prevent it from sticking. Finally, once your sauce is prepared, add pasta to the sauce in a pan and gently warm then plate and serve. This will also ensure that your pasta is not sticky.

Serving portions are generally 50-75g per person for a side dish and 75-100g for a main.

brown butter (beurre noisette)
Melt the butter in a heavy bottomed pan over medium heat whisking until the solids turn brown. The flavour will become nutty. This is used frequently in baking and to give depth of flavour to sauces.

chilli paste and using chillies for seasoning
I have used a chilli sauce for decades called Sriracha which is a 'Sambal Malaysian' variant. It adds more lift and less heat to sauces and marinades. Others are: North African Harissa; Ancho, which is a Mexican variation; and Nam Prik Pao the Thai version made from roasted chillies. Generally, fresh chillies are less intense than dried. If you want full flavour but not so much heat remove the seeds.

clarified butter (ghee)
Put the butter into a heavy-bottomed saucepan and melt over medium heat. Skim off the foam. Carefully pour the clear liquid into a container and discard the whey (white solids).

Clarified butter keeps for several weeks in the refrigerator. It's good for sealing potted dishes and pates and is excellent for frying and basting as it can withstand high temperatures without burning.

croutons
white bread
250ml olive oil
handful of herbs de provençe
salt & pepper

Set oven to broil then cut some white bread or baguette into 1 inch chunks. Next mix oil and seasoning in a bowl. Lightly dip bread into the mixture but do not soak and place on a baking tray. Broil until the croutons are golden, flip them over and return to the grill. This should take no more than a minute per side and be careful because they can burn quickly.

hollandaise

325 ml clarified butter

2 egg yolks

2 tbsp of cold water

1 tbsp of lemon juice

1 tsp of salt

drop of sriracha or pinch of cayenne pepper

In a clean glass bowl, whisk the egg yolks with 2 tbsp of cold water until frothy. Place the bowl over the pan of simmering water and whisk until thickened. Remove from the heat and whisk for a further minute to allow the eggs to cool then place back over the hot water but remove the pan from the heat. Slowly pour the melted butter into the egg yolk mixture continuously whisking. Add the remaining ingredients until they have blended together and the sauce is as thick as you require.

marinades

Marinades have three basic uses. They add flavour, moisture and, in some instances cook meat. This is a way of tenderising lesser cuts of meats. The acids introduced by ingredients such as citrus fruit, wine and vinegars cook meats such as carpaccio. Dry marinades introduce flavour by infusing spices whilst liquid marinades add moisture as well as flavour.

mayonnaise

The type of oil will determine the richness. Use sunflower for light and olive for richer and peppery. This contains raw egg so must be kept refrigerated in a sealed container and used within 2 days.

1 egg yolk,

1 tbsp dijon mustard

salt and freshly cracked black pepper, to taste

200ml oil, sunflower or extra virgin olive oil

juice of 1 lemon, add to taste

Whisk the egg yolk, mustard, salt and pepper until smooth and the salt is dissolved. Then whisk the oil a drop at a time until the mixture begins to emulsify. Continue to add in a steady but delicate stream until thick. Add lemon juice and final seasoning to taste.

mesclun

The term comes from the South of France meaning mixed. It is a combination of young sweet, bitter and spicy leaves including: mizuna; oak leaf lettuce; dandelion; swiss chard; rocket; chervil; mustard greens; beetroot greens; endive and others. It is easily bought pre-packaged in most grocery stores.

pinapple

Cut off the top and bottom and stand on end. A bread knife is a good tool for this. Notice that the 'eyes' run down in columns. Take off the skin in vertical slices, with a column of eyes in the centre, just deep enough to remove them. Follow the shape of the fruit. Remove any leftover eyes then cut in 1 inch thick slices. If not fully ripe the core might be a bit hard and can also be removed.

poaching eggs

Lay a flat plate on the bottom of a skillet to prevent the eggs from sticking. Add enough water for a cracked egg to be submerged in and heat to 80°C. Gently crack and drop in the egg. Cook for a couple minutes until the white is cooked and the yolk is hot but still soft. Remove with a slotted spoon and remove excess moisture on kitchen roll.

preparing rice

There are so many tried and tested techniques. The standard I subscribe to is to soak the rice in cold water (2 parts water to 1 rice) for 10 minutes or rinse for 2-3 minutes in a colander. This removes excess starch. Place the rice in boiling water with a bit of oil and cook for about 10 minutes. The rice should be soft but not mushy. Rinse again in cold water to take out starch and stop the cooking process. Wild and Camargue rice take about double the time to cook.

roux

Mix equal amounts of flour and butter stirring constantly with a wooden spoon over low heat for 5 minutes until the mixture froths a little (the flour must be fully cooked through). Leave to cool until ready to make your sauce.

stock

The two things we usually do not have in home kitchens are time and capacity. Great stock is made over long periods of time and with the refuse of other ingredients, and done in large quantities. Alternatives are readily available. The modern cook can buy any number of pre-prepared stocks – canned, cubed or gels. All are good if you are not a purist. For concentrates and cubes, read the contents and choose one that has stock and meat or vegetable as the main ingredient instead of salt.

vinaigrette

This is based on classic French cookery. To this you can add flavours such as, raspberries, honey or whatever suits your menu.

½ litre olive oil
1 tbsp dry mustard
splash of balsamic vinegar
1 garlic clove, crushed
1 shallot, finely chopped
¼ cup fresh herbs or ⅛ cup herbs de provençe
1 egg yolk
drop of sriracha
salt & pepper

wasabi

Japanese horseradish. It is readily available in pre-made or powdered form from most grocers. Add water and voila!

glossary

arugula – rocket

aubergine – eggplant

bain marie – a pan cotaining hot water that smaller pans are put into to cook slowly

beetroot – beet

Camargue red rice – a nutty wild rice from the Camargue region in the south of France

caster sugar – refined sugar, when using sugar for jellies or other fine desserts where the sugar is melted in liquid, use granulated sugar as it is 'cleaner'

celeriac – celery root

cook without colour – sauté until softened but not browning

coriander – cilantro

crème fraiche – lightly soured cream

double cream – heavy cream

grill – broiler or salamander

herbs de provençe – dried basil, oregano, rosemary, sariette and thyme

Italian tomatoes – roma or pomodoro tomatoes

jelly – gelatine dessert 'jello' or jellied condiment

julienne – finely sliced slivers

Maldon salt – flaked sea salt from east of England. When seasoning raw meats and fish use course salt as fine table salt will leech into the meat

mesclun – a Provençal mixture of sweet and spicy young salad leaves. Traditionally chervil, leafy lettuces and endive. Now frequently added greens are, dandelion, frisee, rocket, mizuna, mach, radicchio, mustard greens and sorrel

parchment – waxed paper

pudding – dessert (in English pudding is a broader term for dessert and also sweet or savoury steamed dishes such as Yorkshire pudding. In America it is usually identified with a sweet creamy dessert)

pumpkin – squash

season to taste – salt & pepper

spring onions – green onions or scallions (a larger version)

stock – broth

tomato purée – tomato paste

tenderloin – fillet

wasabi – Japanese horseradish (can usually be bought in a paste or powdered form)

wild mushrooms – includes chanterelles, chestnut, field, penny bun, porcini, trompette and japanes

Index

A

alcohol 11
allium – garlic, onions,
  - leek & chives 18
angel hair ragu 138
apple
  - & rhubarb crumble 250, 251
  - baked, & cinnamon
    ice cream 258
Asian vegetables, sautéed 160, 161
asperagus wrapped in prosciutto
  with melon 156, 157
artichoke, globe, with lemon
  mayo 158
avocado 18
  - guacamole 63
  - prawn &, cocktail 70, 71

B

bacon & egger 28, 29
bbq salsa 62
bean 18
  - broad, pesto 132
  - French & onion ring casserole
     165
  - legumes and pulses 18
  - puy lentils & shallots 150
  - refried pinto 150
  - Tuscan, soup 96, 97
  - white, sausage & kale soup
     86, 87
beef
  - bourguignon 228, 229
  - cabbage rolls 238, 239
  - medallions of Aberdeen angus
     & mushroom duxelle 230
  - rich Russian borscht 93
  - teriyaki brochettes 244, 245
  - warm, salad with raspberries
     232, 233
beetroot 18
  - & horseradish salad 110
  - chocolate, & tart 260, 261
  - creamy risotto 140, 141
  - rich Russian borscht 92, 93
  - roasted, & goat's cheese salad
     118, 119
berries 19
  - blueberry & yoghurt whippie
     36, 37

  - very berry breakfast smoothie
     28
biscotti 268
boiling pasta 280
bok choi (cruciferous vegetables)
     19
bread
  - cheese straws 58, 59
  - croutons 280
  - italian stuffed 52, 53
  - pitta toasties 60, 61
  - pizza dough 124
  - zucchini 276, 277
broccoli (cruciferous vegetables) 19
  - puree 166
brownies, auntie winona's 259
brussels sprouts (cruciferous
  vegetables) 19
butter
  - brown 280
  - clarified (ghee) 280
  - wasabi 188

C

cabbage (cruciferous vegetables)
     19
  - ichiban slaw 111
  - rolls 238, 239
carrots 19
courgette
  - Brittany 156, 157
  - stuffed globe 155
casseroles
  - French bean & onion ring 165
  - slow roast pheasant 214, 215
  - tuna 131
cauliflower (cruciferous vegetables)
     19
  - cream of &, cumin soup 94
caviar
  - smoked salmon &, blinis 64
  - smoked alaskan salmon &,
     fettuccini 128, 129
cesar salad 102, 103
cheese
  - goat's cheese
     - & chestnut crumble tart
       54, 55
     - & marinated pepper crostini
       65

  - roasted beetroot &, salad
     118, 119
  - soufflé 42, 43
  - straws 58, 59
  - Welsh rarebit 66, 67
chestnut
  - goat's cheese &, crumble tart
     54, 55
  - soup 76, 77
chicken
  - Buffalo wings 212, 213
  - coq au vin 204, 205
  - enchiladas 216-218
  - garam masala 219
  - leek & mushroom chasseur 206
  - liver parfait 56, 57
  - provencal lemon 208
chilli sauce & paste (sriracha)
     11, 208, 209
chive (allium) 18
chocolate
  - & banana smoothie 35
  - & beetroot tart 260, 261
  - crème de menthe &, frippery 65
  - silk pie 264, 265
  - rum truffles 263
cobb salad 115
courgette
  - Brittany 166, 167
  - stuffed globe 155
couscous, tabouleh 104
crepes 47
croutons 280
cruciferous vegetables 19

D

drinks
  - frozen grapes in juice 30, 31
  - fruit juice cubes in yoghurt 31
  - pineapple & ginger sherbet
     32, 33
duck
  - breast of, in tamari marinade
     207
  - crispy, pancakes 220, 221

E

egg
  - bacon & egger 28, 29
  - savoury, cupcakes 45

- organic & egg yolk 19
- poached, with beans on toast 41
- poaching method 282
- quails 68
- salad 114
- cheese soufflé 42, 43

F
fennel
- Mediterranean, salad 105
- pastis prawns on braised 198, 199
fish
- haddock, smoked with pea & baby leek risotto 142, 143
- lemon sole & salsa 194, 195
- pie 192, 193
- salmon
  - smoked Alaskan salmon & caviar fettuccini 128, 129
  - smoked & caviar blinis 64
  - wild native Canadian 178, 179
- sardines, grilled with wasabi butter 188, 189
- sea bass, baked with cepes 182
- trout fillets with tomatoes, ginger & lemongrass 197
- tuna
  - carpaccio 196
  - casserole 131
  - salad 114
  - seared with green curry sauce 184-186
flaxseed (oily fish &) 20
french toast 40

G
garlic (alliums) 18
ginger
- onion roasted with 153
- pinapple &, sherbet 32, 33
- prawn &, soup 78, 79
goat's cheese
- & chestnut crumble tart 54, 55
- roasted beetroot &, salad 118, 119
grapes frozen with juice 30, 31
greek salad 106, 107

guacamole 63

H
hollandaise sauce 281
horseradish
- beetroot &, salad 110
- hummus & pita toasties 60, 61

I
ice lollies, gin & tonic 262
ichiban slaw 111
Italian stuffed bread 52, 53

J
jalapenos (peppers &) 20
jelly, champagne 272, 273

K
kale (cruciferous vegetables) 19
- white bean, sausage &, soup 86, 87

L
lamb
- keema kaleji 240, 241
- simon's pie 234, 235
- welsh cawl 242, 243
leek (allium) 18
- creamy cheesy
- potato & pottage
legumes (beans, & pulses) 18
lemon
- limoncello gelato 270
- loaf 256, 257
- posset 270
- tart 274, 275

M
macaroni, dijon & four cheese 136, 137
mango, smoothie 32
marinades 10, 281
mayonnaise 281
measurement conversion 278
melba toast 68
mesclun 281
mushroom 19
- cepes 68
- cream of, soup & herb crostini 95

- duxelle 68, 164, 260
- pappardelle in truffle cream trompette 222
- wild, & truffle cream
- pappardelle 135
- wild, tart 69

N
nuts (seeds &) 20

O
oily fish 20
okra, roasted 154
old fashioned French toast 40
omega 3 (oily fish & flaxseed) 20
onion (allium) 18
- caramelised, & truffle pizza 127
- roasted with ginger 153
- sage, sweetcorn &, chowder 84, 85
oven temperatures 279

P
partridge cock-a-leekie soup 82
pastry 10
pavlova 226, 227
pears, caramelised with cardamom 252, 253
penne pesto 130
pepper (spices) 10, 21
peppers
- & jalapenos 20
- marinated, & goat's cheese crostini 65
pesto
- basil & pinenut 130
- broad bean 132
petit pois & pearl onions, French style 162
pheasant, slow roast casserole 214, 215
pineapple
- & ginger sherbet 32, 33
- frozen grapes in juice 30, 31
- peppered with crème de cacao sauce 271
- preparation 281
pitta toasties 60, 61
pizza
- caramelised onion & truffle 127

- dough   124
- sauce   126
- toppings   126
plum frangipane tart   254, 255
pork, tenderloin piri piri   236
potato
- & leek pottage   33
- dauphinoise   148, 148
- rosti   168, 169
- salad   112, 113
probiotics (yoghurt &)   22
pumpkin, spicy soup   88, 89
pulses (beans - legumes &)   18

Q

quail, roast with celeriac &
trompette   222, 223
quails eggs with mushroom duxell
& hollandaise   68

R

ragu, angel hair   138, 139
rhubarb, apple &, crumble   250, 251
rice
- jasmin coconut   162, 163
- preparation   282
risotto
- creamy beetroot   140, 141
- smoked haddock with pea &
baby leek   142, 143
roux   282

S

sage, sweetcorn & onion chowder
   85
salsa, bbq   63
salt   11
sauce   10
- four cheese & Dijon   137
- green curry   185, 186
- hollandaise   281
- mignonette   191
- mushroom chasseur   206
- pink peppercorn   237
- pizza   126
- ragu   138
seeds   20
shakes   28
- blueberry & yoghurt whippie
   36, 37

- crème de menthe & chocolate
frippery   35
shallot tart   172, 173
shellfish
- clams in cream & cider   183
- crab claw linguini with
french beans & broad bean
pesto   132, 133
- escargot   197
- nova scotia clam chowder
   90, 91
- oysters, popped   190, 191
- prawn
- & avocado cocktail   70, 71
- & ginger soup   78, 79
- pastis, on braised fennel
   198, 199
- scallop, warm salad   180, 181
smoothies
- chocolate banana   35
- mango   32
- very berry breakfast   28, 29
soufflé, cheese   42, 43
spaghetti carbonara   134
spices   21
spinach salad   116, 117
spirits   11
sriracha   11
stock   282
swede, potato &, mash   152, 153

T

tabouleh   104
thai green curry paste   185, 186
tomato   21
tortilla chips   63
truffle
- caramelised onion &, pizza   127
- chocolate rum   263
- wild mushroom pappardelle in,
cream   135
tumeric (spices)   21
turkey, christmas smash   210, 211

V

veal, escallop of, & pink peppercorn
sauce   237
venison, filet of & chocolate jus   231
vinaigrette   282

W

waffles   46
wasabi   282
water   21
watercress (spinach &)   21
- & crispy shallot salad   108, 109
- creamy, soup   80, 81
welsh rarebit   66, 67
white bean, sausage & kale soup   86
wine   11
whole grain   21

Y

yoghurt   22
- smoothies & shakes   28-36
- with fruit juice ice cubes   31
Yorkshire pudding   171

Z

zabaglioni marsala with berries
& biscotti   268, 269
zucchini bread   276, 277